USING NEUROSCIENCE IN TRAUMA THERAPY

Using Neuroscience in Trauma Therapy provides a basic overview of the structure and function of the brain and nervous system, with special emphasis on changes that occur when the brain is exposed to trauma. The book presents a unique and integrative approach that blends soma and psyche beyond the purview of traditional talk therapy and introduces a variety of trauma-informed approaches for promoting resilience. Each chapter includes case studies, examples, and practical and adaptable tools, making *Using Neuroscience in Trauma Therapy* a go-to guide for information on applying lessons from neuroscience to therapy.

Julie A. Uhernik, RN, LPC, NCC, is a clinician in private practice in Colorado. In addition to counseling work with couples, individuals, and families, she specializes in disaster mental health and trauma. She has worked in emergency planning and public health and serves on several national disaster mental health response teams.

USING NEUROSCIENCE IN TRAUMA THERAPY

Creative and Compassionate Counseling

Julie A. Uhernik

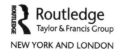

Routledge
Taylor & Francis Group

NEW YORK AND LONDON

First published 2017
by Routledge
711 Third Avenue, New York, NY 10017

and by Routledge
2 Park Square, Milton Park, Abingdon, Oxon, OX14 4RN

Routledge is an imprint of the Taylor & Francis Group, an informa business

Library of Congress Cataloging-in-Publication Data
Names: Uhernik, Julie A., author.
Title: Using neuroscience in trauma therapy : creative and compassionate
    counseling / Julie A. Uhernik.
Description: New York, NY : Routledge, 2016. | Includes bibliographical
    references and index.
Identifiers: LCCN 2016000226 | ISBN 9781138888111 (hbk : alk. paper) |
    ISBN 9781138888128 (pbk. : alk. paper) | ISBN 9781315709710 (ebk)
Subjects: LCSH: Post-traumatic stress disorder—Treatment. | Psychic
    trauma—Treatment. | Neuropsychology.
Classification: LCC RC552.P67 U34 2016 | DDC 616.85/21—dc23
LC record available at http://lccn.loc.gov/2016000226

ISBN: 978-1-138-88811-1 (hbk)
ISBN: 978-1-138-88812-8 (pbk)
ISBN: 978-1-315-70971-0 (ebk)

Typeset in Baskerville
by Apex CoVantage, LLC

Trauma survivors whose courage and strength inspire
The tireless work of colleagues in the trauma trenches
To Dexter—model for unabashed joy

CONTENTS

FIGURES

PREFACE

As a compassionate but somewhat geeky nursing student, I frequently wandered down to the North Dakota State University basement of Sudro Hall, past the pharmacy labs and classrooms, to a long hallway with a row of eye-level shelves. The shelves were lined with specimen jars, large and small. A jar containing a human brain caught my attention. An off-white color, with many wrinkles and folds, the brain was floating eerily in preserving fluid. I recall being fascinated as I looked at it. I wondered about the life of the person whose brain I gazed upon. I wondered about the intricacies of thoughts, of memories, and personal life experiences processed and contained in this floating specimen in front of me.

In nursing class, we were learning the anatomy and function of the brain, how to identify frontal lobe, temporal lobe, corpus callosum, and more. At the same time, my nursing education focused outward, on compassionate caring and the interpersonal support helpful in moments of trauma, illness, and misfortune. My graduate education in counseling further blended this unique mix of the interpersonal caring and inner knowledge, learning, and experience. Clinical practice, as well as mental health responses to disaster, has offered an opportunity to observe and witness the aftermath of trauma, whether common experiences of trauma from disasters or the intimate internal experience of trauma held as memories from long ago. With curiosity, necessity, and feeling overwhelmed, I have read of the latest neuroscience discoveries and of the new findings about the brain, the nervous system, and the intricacies of cellular, genetic, and chemical reactions within brain and body.

We have now the ability to view the brain and its functions in living time. Research is confirming what was long suspected: that the power in healing a wounded brain may come through interpersonal connections and through resilience in the face of whatever environmental circumstances come along. The continuing requirement for learning updates, the wonders of the brain, and the courageous examples of people sorting through trauma is constant inspiration to me.

This book is for counselors, care providers, and the curious, and may provide an easy-to-understand look at the brain, the body, and how integrated therapeutic approaches may provide a gentle nudge toward healing and well-being.

For readers hoping to learn fundamentals about the brain, they will discover everything from the differences between a neurotransmitter and neurohormone, to the migration and clustering of neurons in utero. They will want to check the first four chapters of this book for a review of anatomical and functional aspects of the nervous system. For readers seeking better understanding of neuroscience in light of subjective or even collective experiences of trauma, chapters 5 through 8 will be their go-to location. Chapter 9 suggests new and integrative approaches to trauma treatment. And finally, chapter 10 provides a window into neuroscience discoveries present and future, which may inform, guide, and validate the work of healing the mind.

A few important items of clarification are in order. The term 'client' rather than 'patient' is used most often throughout the book. The intent is to find the best linguistic way to differentiate a person experiencing trauma from the healer, therapist, or guide who is working with him or her. Likewise, this book may use terms such as 'therapist,' 'counselor,' or 'trauma worker' interchangeably. There are case examples scattered throughout the book. Not intended as a clinical process outline or directive pointing toward a particular therapeutic approach, these examples will hopefully illustrate neuroscience connections behind suggested adjuncts to treatments. Composites have been used in case examples along with removal of identifying specifics or details. In some examples, colleagues whose therapeutic orientation and approach may differ from conventional psychotherapeutic approaches have weighed in. For example, included are examples from a clinician who approaches trauma treatment from an energy psychology perspective. There are examples from nurses in the field. There are examples of the treatment focus used in disaster response with population- and community-based interventions. This may, on some level, help all care providers to learn and respect similarities and differences as clinicians, and point to benefits of learning and collaborating without boundaries. These are times of exciting discoveries and for approaching the treatment of trauma and applications of neuroscience with a spirit of collaboration, curiosity, and creativity.

Following ethical guidelines of every therapy discipline, adjuncts to trauma treatments adopted should always prompt the therapist to gain proper training and instruction, and to always remain aware of scope of practice. The early admonition of Hippocrates of *Primum non nocere* (or First do no harm) has particular relevance in working with those impacted by trauma.

Finally, for both healers and trauma survivors, this book begs consideration of the words of poet Rainer Maria Rilke: "Perhaps all the dragons of our lives are princesses who are only waiting to see us once beautiful and brave."

Julie A. Uhernik
December 2015

ACKNOWLEDGMENTS

I was approached to write this book based upon a presentation given at the 2014 American Counseling Association national conference. Many presentation attendees expressed interest in new research discoveries and practice implications of neuroscience. The knowledge base in brain science is growing so rapidly it can be hard to keep up. This book attempts to provide basic neuroscience information together with new research discoveries that may influence future directions in the mental health field. Examining new research findings may give a gentle nudge to counselors and mental health specialists to think outside the box and be open to approaching mental health care in a holistic and collaborative manner. Above all, these are exciting times for professionals in our field.

I would like to thank colleagues John Harder, Valerie Varan, Beverly White, Melissa Moffit, Miriam Vintner, Amy Martin, and others I am privileged to know and work with, for their professional support and their model of acceptance, curiosity, and openness in service to traumatized people. I owe a debt to professionals in the field of holistic nursing who speak out for integration of complementary, alternative, and adjunctive methods of treatment for trauma, and for encouraging collaboration and cooperation between clinicians in all fields. I give a nod to public health and endeavors that bring the neuroscience research on individual trauma out to a population-based focus and that strive for increased cultural understanding of traumatic experience. I want to thank the American Red Cross for the honor and privilege of working in the midst of disaster and the opportunity to observe the resilience of people in the face of trauma.

I am grateful to Mary Lemma for her skills, attention to detail, and can-do spirit when presented with "just one more thing"; to Trish McCall for encouragement and many pep talks; and to Anna Moore and Zoey Peresman at Routledge for suggestions, comments, and editorial guidance. My gratitude to Kelsey Shroyer, Alexandra Buck, and Luke Shroyer for technical assistance and the savvy they shared with this pencil-and-paper kind of gal. I am grateful to Ken for patience, support, and encouragement.

My gratitude to researchers in brain science who provide us science geeks with enough material to ponder and approaches to integrate for many a therapist career.

Finally, gratitude to my clients for courage, determination, and resiliency in the face of suffering and for gently holding and offering up such beautiful delicate representations of hope. Social cognitive neuroscience speaks of attunement and shared activation in the prefrontal cortex between people and their interactions. Simply put, we are best on this journey together.

1

A NEW LOOK AT
THE AMAZING BRAIN

"If our brains were simple enough for us to understand them,
we'd be so simple that we couldn't."

—Ian Stewart, *The Collapse of Chaos:*
Discovering Simplicity in a Complex World

The amazing, astonishing brain. The complexity and work-ings of the brain have fascinated and intrigued humans since ancient times. Archeological evidence has shown that prehistoric people engaged in trepanning, or the cutting of holes in the skull, for unknown purposes. Archeological findings indicate that trepanning was practiced across cul-tures until as recent as 2000 BC. Forensic evidence has shown that some of the ancient recipients of trepanning actual survived what was perhaps a primitive form of brain sur-gery. While Aristotle focused on the heart as the seat of rea-son, and thought the brain was simply a cooling device that supported the heart, he nevertheless identified brain tasks such as differences in short-term versus long-term memory functions. Later, Romans such as Galen focused more on the ventricles, or spaces deep within the brain, than on the spongy brain material itself. In Renaissance times, Leon-ardo da Vinci, working through autopsy, observed and diagrammed the brain, particularly the optic nerve and pathways, with remarkable precision. It is only in recent times that the branch of science known as neuroscience has begun, along with amazing technological advances, to give us a remarkable understanding of the brain, the nervous system, and the intricate workings that make us who we are. Current findings in the field of neuroscience are helping us understand and provide treatment for trauma and maladies of the brain, body, and functioning.

In April 2013, a new initiative and program was proposed by President Barack Obama to open and encourage research into the brain. Like its research counterpart, the Human Genome Project, this initiative promises to be equally rich in providing fundamental and expansive knowledge of the workings of the human brain. Called the BRAIN (Brain Research through Advancing Innovative Neurotechnologies) Initiative, it seeks to provide understanding of disorders of the brain such as depression, Alzheimer's, and autism and to "deepen our understanding of how we think, learn, and remember" (Obama, 2014).

One wonders if ancient peoples made a connection between processes of thought and the subjective experiences and interpretation of trauma. Fear and trepidation existed around unexplainable neurological conditions such as epilepsy, paralysis, and stroke. These maladies were often approached with supernatural explanations, placing blame on evil spirits, or unexplained 'humors' or liquids supposedly residing in the ventricles of the brain. Current descriptions of effects of trauma on the brain are built on a progression of discoveries and, with each discovery, on a foundation of curiosity and wonder. A prevailing explanation of modern-day reactions to trauma and stress go something like this: *Danger or threat is initially detected through the senses . . . bodies (and minds) are primed to fight, flee, and hopefully to survive in the face of ancient dangers (examples given usually includes a saber-toothed tiger) . . . yet in modern times there is seldom a specific episodic danger (at least not the saber-toothed tiger) . . . just low-level, ongoing perceptions and interpretations of danger that create physiological responses in brain and body.* That explanation, taken along with studies in comparative psychology, points to current understanding of trauma responses in animals and humans. This understanding has influenced recent work around trauma, with many contributing researchers studying the brain and the body in adaptation to stress.

New discoveries of brain functioning are occurring daily, as new technologies become available to study the brain in real time and functioning (Raichle, 1998). As scientific discoveries increase, parallel efforts to use new information in clinical ways are also increasing. New technology such as functioning magnetic resonance imaging enables researchers to observe the ongoing response and activity of the various areas of the brain like never seen before. In continued use since 1924, the electroencephalograph and other formats measuring electrical activity of the brain have produced new areas of knowledge to assist in understanding brain function in real time, rather than viewing brain pathology only after death at autopsy. Clinicians and behavioral health specialists face a task of keeping up-to-date on this information explosion and in bringing implications of findings to use. Neuroscience findings can provide assistance to those suffering with mental illness, traumatic experiences, and life events and can help people become resilient, adaptable, and content in face of vicissitudes of life.

Recent Advances in Brain Imaging

In 1924, German psychiatrist Hans Berger discovered that signals of electrical activity in the brain could be detected by placing electrode sensors over the scalp. Known as an electroencephalograph, or EEG, this enabled doctors to pinpoint areas of increased electrical activity within the brain (see Figure 1.1).

Normal Adult Brain Waves

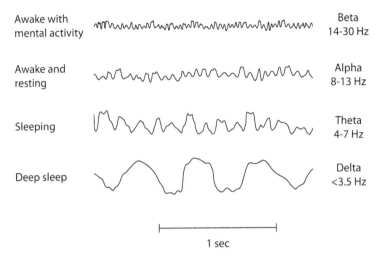

Figure 1.1 EEG—Electrical Activity in Brain

Communication between neurons proceeds through means of electrical and chemical conduction. EEG has allowed researchers to observe common electrical patterns seen in normal functioning, including the electrical activity in the brain during alert, waking states and the electrical pulses of the brain during sleep. In the 1960s, research out of UCLA led to advances in EEG technology and introduced computer digital analysis of brain functioning known as quantitative EEG (QEEG). Through QEEG, mapping of brain functions and comparison with normative data became available to the clinician.

Another method of visualizing the brain and surrounding tissues was also developed in the 1920s. Called cerebral angiography, it measured blood flow through the arteries and veins within the brain, which is seen as an indirect indicator of the level of oxygenation to the brain. Cerebral angiography works by injecting a contrast agent or dye into the carotid artery in the neck and then following the dye by X-ray as it circulates through the blood vessels and throughout the brain. Cerebral angiography has allowed doctors to detect blood vessel malformations, aneurysm, or the damage to areas of the brain affected by stroke. Cerebral angiography may also point to blood vessels that appear out of place, which may be an indicator of a collected blood supply to feed a fast-growing brain tumor.

In the early 1990s, neuroscience research advanced rapidly through the use of magnetic resonance imaging (MRI). Like angiography in some ways, MRI also works by measuring local changes in blood volume of the brain, and indicates levels of oxygenation to areas of the brain. Specifically, MRI examines the red blood cell concentration, and because red blood cells contain an iron-rich hemoglobin molecule, blood concentration can be detected through the magnetic pulses applied through the MRI machine (see Figure 1.2).

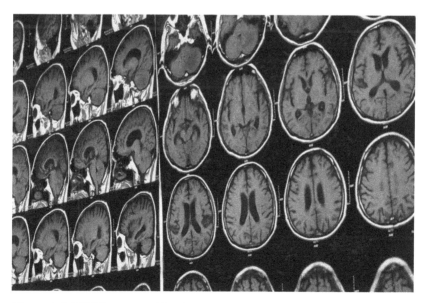

Figure 1.2 MRI Images of Brain

The MRI can pick up local changes in blood volume in the brain. This imaging technique gives a clear digital picture of the structures of the brain, appearing as though looking through many slices of brain sections. The technology of MRI was used initially as a tool for diagnosis. In the early 1990s, what is known as functional MRI (fMRI) began to be used for the purpose of understanding how the brain functions. Researchers found that during MRI scanning, brain responses of research participants can be measured in real time. This provides a moving picture of areas of the brain in response to stimuli such as touch and sound, creating so-called activation maps. Activation maps point to areas of activity in various parts of the brain during various mental activities. fMRIs can then take the two-dimensional imagery of an MRI and gather the composite data to create a three-dimensional image. An advantage of using MRI for patients is that it is a noninvasive procedure; for this reason it is frequently used in current neuroscience research.

Newer in the brain imaging field are SPECT scans, or single photon emission computerized tomography, which is a highly specific type of positron emission tomography (PET) scanning. This technology includes a functional imaging technique using small amounts of radioactive substances injected into the body, which are detected as the radioisotope containing a sugar tracer is taken up in active areas of brain associated with glucose metabolism. The result is a clear three-dimensional-appearing brain picture, which when compared to images of healthy brains can indicate possible areas of dysfunction. This technology is very expensive and not available in many places. In addition, the technology exposes the patient to radiation, which can limit the advisability of repeated scans and further radiation exposure.

The descriptions of the newest imaging techniques begin to sound as if they are out of a science fiction or futuristic novel. Magnetoencephalography (MEG) is a noninvasive brain imaging method that uses small recording devices called SQUIDS (super conducting quantum interface devices) that detect rapid changes in brain activity through magnetic detection, at the basic neural level, showing activation in cortex areas of the brain in real time. Other recent neuroscience and technological discoveries are focusing upon deeper understanding of neuron functioning and neuron interconnection at the basic cellular level. In 2004, German scientist Winfreid Denk developed an updated version of the electron microscope. Together with the work of other noted scientists, microscopic observation of neurons and groups of neurons is occurring using these new versions of electron microscopy (Denk & Horstmann, 2004). Research is now focusing on the discovery of bundles of neurons and on the interconnection of groups of neurons. These discoveries have brought together researchers, beginning in 2009, for a cooperative project known as the Human Connectome Project. This project aims to map and compile advanced electron microscopic data and proceed to study these interconnected bundles of neurons known as connectomes (Seung, 2012). Chapter 2 will discuss the intriguing research around connectomes in greater detail.

The implications of these and many more neuroscience discoveries will likely change, perhaps confirm, and certainly influence new methods for treatment with trauma-impacted clients.

One of the most interesting and encouraging discoveries in neuroscience is of the capacity of the brain to heal, to repair, and to recover functioning after damage. Called neuroplasticity, this ability to grow and heal has been observed at the level of individual neuronal synapses as well as in entire areas of the brain that reroute following injury to regain and continue functions. A definition of neuroplasticity is "the capacity of the nervous system to develop new neuronal connections" ("Neuroplasticity," n.d.). The concept of neuroplasticity, and the demonstrated capacity of the brain to heal and grow, is guiding clinicians in new treatment directions and providing a support for the efficacy of therapy. Until recently, it was thought that the capacity for brain growth and development was completed at an early age, and that after this period of rapid brain growth, the brain does not change structurally. Early theorists such as William James began to challenge this static view of the brain, but his assumptions were overlooked at the time. In the late 1940s, Canadian psychologist Donald Hebb was studying neural networks within the brain and learning processes (Hebb, 1949). Hebb is credited with the concept that "neurons that fire together, wire together" (although this descriptive expression was actually introduced later by scientist Michael Merzenich; Doidge, 2007). Hebb extended this notion to an explanation of learning processes. Hebb believed that when two connecting neurons repeatedly fire messages one to another, the two neurons both undergo chemical changes that serve to strengthen the connection and increase the impulse activity between both. Current research into neuroplasticity has found that these connected neurons also become faster and more efficient at processing. Further, this ability of neurons to connect and form new neural pathways is present throughout the life span, not just in the rapid brain growth periods of infancy and early childhood. The aforementioned connectome research uses basic Hebbian concepts as a springboard for neuroscience discoveries around functioning networks of neurons.

Current neuroscience research is focusing in the area of neurogenesis. Neurogenesis is defined simply as the formation of nervous tissue ("Neurogenesis," n.d.). Neurogenesis research has discovered that new functioning neurons can be developed from neural stem cells. This process of neurogenesis continues throughout the life span and occurs in certain areas of the brain, primarily the hippocampus. The hippocampus is heavily involved in learning and memory processes (Ming & Song, 2011). Research into neurogenesis is seeking to answer questions about the possibility of the brain regrowing and rewiring following injury, and about reorganization and optimal functioning of the brain throughout a lifetime. Such research continues to inform us about the human experience and the impact and nature of trauma upon the functioning brain, and point to new treatments and support.

References

Denk, W., & Horstmann, H. (2004). Serial block-face scanning electron microscopy to reconstruct three-dimensional tissue nanostructure. *PLoS Biology*, 2(11), e329. http://doi.org/10.1371/journal.pbio.0020329 (retrieved December 2015 from www.ncbi.nlm.nih.gov/pmc/articles/PMC524270/)

Doidge, N.D. (2007). *The brain that changes itself: Stories of personal triumph from the frontiers of brain science.* New York: Penguin Books.

Hebb, D.O. (1949). *The organization of behavior: A neuropsychological theory.* New York: John Wiley & Sons (pg. 62).

Ming, G., & Song, H. (2011). Neurogenesis in the adult mammalian brain: Significant answers and significant questions. *Neuron*, 70(4), 687–702. (retrieved May 11, 2015 from ncbi.nlm.nih.gov)

Neurogenesis. (n.d.). In *The American heritage Stedman's medical dictionary.* (retrieved March 29, 2016 from www.dictionary.com/browse/neurogenesis)

Neuroplasticity. (n.d.). In *Dictionary.com unabridged.* (retrieved March 28, 2016 from www.dictionary.com/browse/neuroplasticity)

Obama, B. (2014, September 30). Brain initiative. (retrieved March 31, 2016 from www.whitehouse.gov/share/brain-initiative)

Raichle, M.E. (1998, February). Behind the scenes of functional brain imaging: A historical and physiological perspective. *Proceedings of the National Academy of Science USA*, 95, 765–772.

(retrieved March 31, 2016 from http://coewww.rutgers.edu/classes/bme/bme450/introduction/raichle98%20765.pdf)

Seung, S. (2012). *Connectome: How the brain's wiring makes us who we are.* New York: Houghton Mifflin Harcourt Publishing Company.

2

BASIC BRAIN FUNCTIONING

In order to understand how the brain responds to environmental circumstances and to internal experience, a simplified overview of the brain and brain functioning is in order.

The amazing complexity of the brain is immediately apparent with the use of new technologies and research into brain functioning. New discoveries in neuroscience are requiring constant update of understanding and implications. Partial credit should be given, however, to thousands of years of curiosity about who we are and to earlier contributions in understanding this cauliflower lookalike encased under our skull. As we consider the inner workings of the brain, we are using the very brain functions we are seeking to understand. It is amazing to possess the perceptual ability and capacity required to observe these inner workings of the brain. We are our own case study. In daily experience, we give little ongoing thought to neural connections and processes at work when we walk across the room with poise and balance, or enjoy the sensory experience of a rose; instead, we simply bask in awareness.

At one level, we have much in common with other vertebrate and invertebrate animals on earth; however, humans, through evolutionary processes, have developed and added functioning layers to the brain. Brain development set the stage for the innovation and advancement of humanity at astonishing rates. Human brain size, particularly as measured in relation to body size, has been thought to be related to a high level of intelligence. In comparing human brains to those of other animals, factors such as the amount of folds within the brain, the amount of gray matter proportional to white matter, and the neuron number and interconnections with other neurons are also important to consider. New findings in the study of genetics are pointing to genome similarities among animals possessing higher level cognitive functioning such as humans, dolphins, and elephants.

However, even the lowly paramecium, a primitive single-celled animal, has a rudimentary nervous system that allows it to move, explore, and interact with its environment.

Anatomy of the Brain and Nervous System

The brain is not the largest functioning organ in the human body—that distinction goes to our skin—but the brain is certainly one of the most complex. Weighing around three pounds, it sits in the cranial cavity, floating and cushioned in protective fluid. It appears whitish in color, yet contains what is referred to as gray matter and white matter. White matter of the brain consists of the many supporting cells, called glial cells, which provide a matrix surrounding the gray matter, which is made up of neurons. The brain is richly supplied with blood vessels that carry oxygen-rich blood to the brain. These blood vessels also bring a continuing supply of glucose to meet the vast energy needs of the brain. In fact, although the brain consists of just 2% of the weight of the body, it requires 20% of the glucose (energy) demands of the body. Deprivation of either oxygen or glucose can result in irreparable damage to the brain within 10 minutes. Brain tissue deprived of oxygen begins to decompose within those 10 minutes. Depriving the brain of a steady level of glucose leads to increasing reactivity and ultimate instability of cellular functioning. For example, in a diabetic, fluctuating blood glucose levels can result in initial irritability and mood changes. If a blood glucose level drops too low without the administration of or intake of a source of glucose, the brain will respond with eventual shutdown including seizure, coma, and then death.

The brain sits within the skull as if surrounded by an upside-down bowl. The brain is covered with three layers of membranes called meninges, which line the skull and provide an extra layer of cushion between brain and skull. The brain can be thought to float in this upside-down, hard-sided bowl of the skull. It is bathed in cerebrospinal fluid, which helps to cushion and protect the brain by absorbing shock from blows to the head. Current research attention is focused on damage to the brain from head injury or what is commonly called traumatic brain injury (TBI). While results from TBI can be immediately life threatening, subtle neural damage from even mild injury may also occur. For example, recent findings point to an association between head injury and an increase in risky behaviors in adolescents (Thompson, 2014). In a 2008 research review by Schwarzbold et al., the association of TBI to various psychiatric disorders is discussed. Of special interest to trauma clinicians, any subsequent development of PTSD (post-traumatic stress disorder), mood disorders and cognitive impairments following history of head injury should be explored and considered as a routine part of clinical evaluation and assessment. The frontal lobe of the brain appears to be particularly vulnerable to damage from head injury. Damage to the frontal lobe can negatively affect decision making and executive planning, with resulting increase in risky behaviors (McKee & Robinson, 2014). New information is available for clinicians supporting education for prevention of head injury and on assessment of, and treatment for, damage to the brain due to head trauma. Counselors and other mental health specialists should include in every intake assessment an inquiry of history of head traumas and concussions.

The brain has many convolutions and folds, mostly seen within the outer area of the cerebrum. These folds allow for a larger brain surface area than is readily apparent on simple examination. The folds and convolutions allow the brain to fit snuggly inside the skull. These folds extend lengthwise from the head down to the upper area of the spinal column. The brain contains inner ventricles or chambers that are filled with constantly replenished cerebral spinal fluid. Cerebral spinal fluid carries nutrients to the brain and removes waste products from the brain.

Recent medical attention is focused on the importance of identifying and treating head injuries. Many returning war veterans have suffered head injuries during their service, and increasing brain-related injuries are noted in sports and some workplace environments. Recent high-profile cases in the NFL have pointed to connections between repeated concussions and brain injury and the later development of chronic traumatic encephalopathy as noted upon autopsy of former players (Gavett et al., 2011). There is a great need for education, identification, and prevention of head injury and trauma.

Counselors and trauma-focused therapists may assist their clients to connect with medical resources for head trauma treatment and to develop collaborative treatment planning. Often, clients themselves do not associate past injuries as relevant to current mental health status and functioning. A trauma-aware counselor will inquire about history of head or spinal injuries, gain a complete diagnostic picture, and assist in treatment planning and problem solving with head injury awareness.

The brain sits at the top of the body, acting as a director and coordinator of activity and action throughout the body. It does so through nerves located in the brain and through nerves that extend down through the spinal cord and outward to the body. There are 31 pairs of spinal nerves that branch out to all parts of the body. Within the head, there are also 12 pairs of cranial nerves, which are linked directly within the brain and the brain stem. The cranial nerves primarily connect to the sensory organs (eye, ear, and nose) and provide enervation for important movements such as chewing, speaking, and eye movements. Cranial nerves are responsible for minute and intricate movements involved in facial expressions, to which humans respond and with which they interact, fostering an all-important social connection. The vagus nerve is the longest cranial nerve and has the most cranial branches. It is intricately involved in autonomic nervous system regulation. An understanding of vaso–vagal nerve responses and influences on body organs such as heart, lungs, muscles, and digestive system leads to a discussion of sympathetic and parasympathetic nervous system responses. The vagus nerve plays a key role in the functioning of the autonomic nervous system, which is crucial to body maintenance functions, as well as to the body's responses to stress and environmental stimuli. In Chapter 3 we will learn of the vagal nerve pathway and specific implications of this important neural pathway for the trauma-informed counselor.

It is helpful to consider the brain as having three functioning layers from the base of the brain to the top of the head. The brain is further divided into two hemispheres, one on the right side of the skull and one on the left, and these hemispheres are connected by a structure called the corpus callosum. The corpus callosum allows for communication between the neurons in both brain hemispheres. The cerebral cortex, with its many folds and convolutions, wraps around the sides and over the top area of the brain. For purposes of location and identification, specific regions of the cerebral cortex are identified as lobes, or specialized areas. The right and left hemisphere are roughly symmetrical and include the same areas or lobes on each side (see Figure 2.1). These lobes include the frontal lobe, parietal lobe, and temporal lobe. In the rear portion of the brain, at the back of the head, is the occipital lobe. The cerebellum is located underneath the occipital lobe, in the back lower area of the head. Interestingly, the cerebrum of the brain makes up 85% of the total weight of the brain while the cerebellum makes up approximately 10% of the brains' total weight. The brain stem is located deep and center at the base of the brain, just above the spinal cord. Brain lobes correspond somewhat loosely with different areas of functionality in the brain. For example, located within the parietal lobe(s), sitting atop and across the back of the head, are areas that include direction of physiological functions for the orientation of the body in space, and the functions

ANATOMY OF THE BRAIN

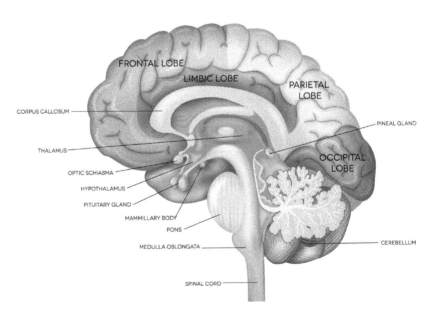

Figure 2.1 Anatomy of the Brain

of attention, alertness and focus. Counselors, in seeking to provide a simple anatomical explanation to clients of functional cortical areas of the brain, can illustrate location by making an 'L' shape with the index finger and thumb and superimposing it onto the side of the skull, with the tip of the index finger near midline pointing up and the thumb pointing sideways toward the ear. The counselor can then indicate functionality of areas of the cortex. To illustrate a rough three-dimensional model of the brain, the counselors can raise their hand with palm facing outward, placing the thumb along the inside of the palm. The counselor can point out that the thumb represents the inner limbic system of the brain. Then, upon closing the fingers over and making a fist, can explain how the cortex is wrapped over the top of the brain. The brain stem can be pointed to as the wrist area, and extending down the arm is the spinal cord (Siegel, 2010). While simplistic, such illustrations can be helpful for clients as they gain basic understanding of brain responses to and recovery from trauma.

Viewing the brain from underneath, one would see a portion of the frontal lobe and temporal lobe on the right and left side, as well as the olfactory bulb leading from the nose, the pons and cerebellum, and the 12 cranial nerves. The internal parts of the brain are usually viewed from a sagittal (or vertical) view, often by dividing down the corpus callosum and looking from inside to out. Major structures seen in this manner would include the cingulate sulcus, diencephalon, anterior commissure, and temporal lobe portions. From this viewpoint, one would also see the midbrain, containing the limbic system structures of the amygdala, hypothalamus, and hippocampus, and below it the pons, cerebellum, and the poetically named medulla oblongata. It is thought that the human brain and nervous system evolved in a bottom-up fashion, sharing the early gestational development patterns of other vertebrates. Over time, the human brain greatly increased in the amount of the area and density of the cerebral cortex. This increase in cortical area is a contributing factor to human development and advancement of higher level reasoning and functional skills.

The Neuron and Mighty Network

If we zero in on brain tissue with a microscope, we can narrow down to a view of a single nerve cell known as a neuron. Neurons, the defining cells of the nervous system, are unique in shape in the cellular world. All neurons contain a cell body with a nucleus that contains DNA, mitochondria that supply energy to the neuron, and other cellular parts necessary for the functioning and maintenance of the cell. Extending away from the neuron like a branch is the axon, which serves as a connector to other neurons, passes along information, and includes upwards of 100,000 dendrites (like miniature branches). The close proximity of dendrites and their connections to other neurons make up the primary pathway through which neurons communicate. Dendrites can be thought of as tiny receivers of information at the ends or extensions of the neuron. There are a number of variations on this basic neuron configuration, which may include a unipolar neuron with one axon leading away from the nucleus and then dividing into two axon 'terminals,' bipolar neurons with one set of dendrite extensions and axon extension, or the most common type of neuron, called a multipolar neuron, which has many sets of dendrites and one main axon (see Figure 2.2).

A single neuron may hold the distinction of being the longest type of cell in the body. Such a neuron may run along the length of the spinal cord and along the sensory or motor neuron pathways. These lengthy neurons are no less impressive however, than a shorter neuron, each having an

Different kinds of neurons

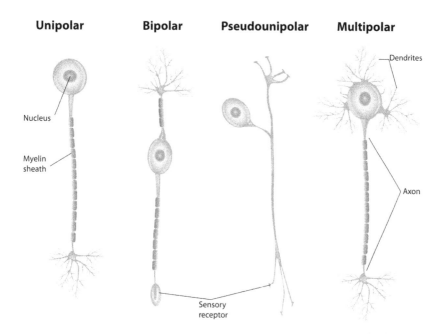

Unipolar   **Bipolar**   **Pseudounipolar**   **Multipolar**

Dendrites

Nucleus

Myelin
sheath

Axon

Sensory
receptor

Figure 2.2 Types of Neurons

astounding number of connections and capacity for receiving and processing information. This number of possible connections is estimated to be more than the number of atoms in the universe. The interconnections of neurons to other neurons results in the possibility of an estimated 100 trillion connections. As amazing as individual neurons are, their actions and functions would not exist without space between these neural points of connections. These spaces are called synapses. The actions that occur in the synaptic space can be functionally divided into two concepts. First, there is the concept of divergence, where a message sent out from one neuron can affect numerous other neurons. Second, there is convergence, where a single neuron can simultaneously receive input signals from many other cells.

Neural cellular development, beginning just after conception, is all about a journey. An amazing neuron production process takes place during human gestation. During peak months of fetal development, an estimated 250,000 neurons are being produced each minute (LeDoux, 2002). Initially, some of the divided cells located on the outside of the blastocyst (the bundle of cells growing just after fertilization) begin to migrate toward an inner cluster of the developing cells, almost like folding in on itself, moving to the inside of the ball of cells. These cells begin to form something akin to a tube with the rudimentary formation of a future brain located on one end, and the tube extending the length to the other end. Running along this length of neurons is the early formation of the spinal cord and peripheral nerves. From earliest moments after conception, cells are dividing and continue to divide at a rapid and furious pace. By the eighth week, the brain itself has developed into its three regions, the forebrain, midbrain, and hindbrain. In the early weeks there are an estimated 250,000 neuroblasts, the primitive precursors to neurons. Neural production begins around gestational day 42, and neurons immediately begin a process of migration to various areas of the brain. In this manner, basic neural pathways are complete at birth (Stiles & Jernigan, 2010) Initially, there is a vast overproduction of neuroblasts to help with the enormous task of establishing connection networks. Neurons that strengthen their connection together grow and thrive, while large numbers of neurons that don't have strong connections are pruned away.

Neurons that Fire Together Wire Together

From the earliest beginning, nerves cells are about connection and network. It is as though nerve cells reach out to each other from the start, with those cells that connect with other neurons humming with life; those not able to connect will die or be pruned away. Neurons begin the process of a great migration to align with and connect to other neurons. They are helped along the way by other nervous system cells called glial cells. Glial cells provide a lattice-like support, similar to scaffolding, for the neurons as they migrate to various areas throughout the brain (see Figure 2.3).

The glial cells also protect and nourish the neurons, with one type of glial cell that controls neuron cell metabolism and another type of glial cell that coats the neuron with a substance called myelin, forming a sheath-like cover surrounding the neuron, much like the rubber coating around electrical wiring. The presence of myelin controls the speed of conduction of electrical impulses traveling through the axons of neurons. Myelination of neurons and

NEURONS AND NEUROGLIAL CELLS

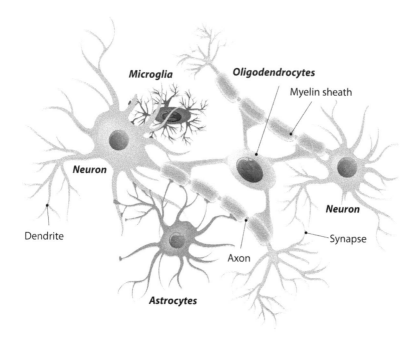

Figure 2.3 Illustration of Glial Cell

impulse conduction problems are implicated in disease processes like multiple sclerosis.

Continuing studies of fetal neuron migration have shown that there are chemical signals called trophic factors that seem to direct neural axons on where to connect. These chemical signals, along with sustained electrical stimulation, determine if the connection between neurons will hold, and ultimately whether a given neuron will survive or die. Because of the vast overproduction of neurons, many of the neural axons are not able to adequately connect and either wither or are pruned away, and the remaining molecules of the cells are recycled. During this time of fetal development, neural cells are developing into cells that will perform different functions, a process called 'differentiation'. These cells begin a migration outward to different parts of the brain; for example, a visual neuron may migrate to the visual cortex area—located in the occipital lobe, or back lower part of the head—or it may join other visual neurons to form the optic nerve. There is evidence that some neurons travel faraway and set up new clusters of neural neighborhoods that in turn open further communications between various neural sites. As neurons connect, the factor of environment comes into play in the form of learning. Visual neurons are stimulated when presented with light and begin a 'learning' process of adapting to and detecting the presence or absence of environmental light. Neural connections that are repeatedly activated by sensory input become stronger, with their connection network staying intact. Neurons without stimulation and connections to other neurons are pruned off.

The common saying that "neurons that fire together wire together" serves to explain this process. The term 'plasticity' refers to the discovered ability of the brain as a whole to change its structure and function. It had long been thought that the structure and functioning capacity of the brain was unchanging after early development was complete. It is now known that brain tissue can be strengthened and can restructure itself in response to learning.

New research is focused on the study of these groups of neurons as they form interconnected networks called connectomes (see Figure 2.4). A connectome is a cluster of

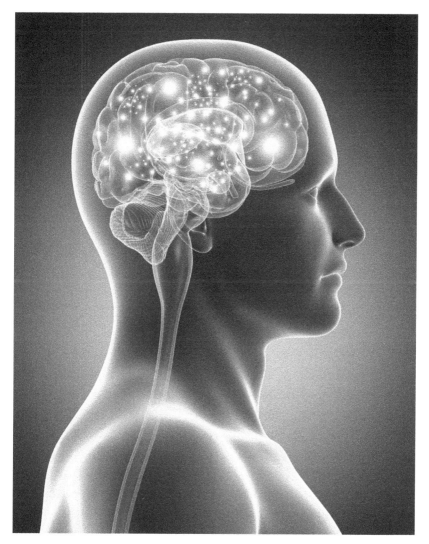

Figure 2.4 Illustration of Neural Connections

synaptic connections where neurons that increasingly signal out to each other, cluster together, and then strengthen and create strong bonds with each other.

Previously, it was thought that each developing fetal cell had a specific functional assignment to migrate toward and a specific location to settle into and that ultimately, when these neural cells combined with other like cells, they would together form all the segments of the entire adult brain. It's now known that many factors can disrupt or alter the migration, which in itself can affect brain development and subsequent functioning. There are many practical implications of these findings leading to new support and preventive efforts to promote healthy development in the early prenatal period of life. This is pointing to renewed interest in and important emphasis upon good maternal and fetal health in the prenatal, birth, and perinatal periods. Maternal state of health, use of substances, hormonal influences, and cellular metabolism are just several possible factors that can have profound effects on neural migration and the subsequent neural connections of the developing fetus. Disorders such as autism, schizophrenia, epilepsy, and others are now thought to have beginnings within faulty migration patterns of neurons in the brain (Ratey, 2001).

The entire brain is itself aligned in a vertical fashion, beginning at the base or brain stem, through the midbrain, and upward toward the cerebral cortex. This alignment is both structural and functional. For example, the functional tasks of the lower brain stem include basic physiological functions such as respiration, while upper areas of the cerebral cortex are focused on functions of learning and problem solving. There is also side-to-side function, with the right hemisphere and left hemisphere connected via the corpus callosum. It is thought that the human brain organized bottom to top during evolution in a similar fashion to what happened with other animal species. Reptiles, birds, and fish, for example, have rudimentary brain stems. The brain stem appears like a widening area at the end of the stalk-like spinal cord. The lower end of the brain stem is situated through an opening in the base of the skull, and its upper area sits at about eye level in the center of the head. The brains of mammals evolved to include midbrain areas such as the limbic system, with the cortex sitting above. Human brain evolution dramatically increased the size, the density, and the convolutions within the cortex, especially in the area of the frontal lobe of the brain.

The brain stem contains the lower brain areas connecting with the spinal cord, the midbrain area, and the lower hind-brain area. At the lowest end of the brain stem sits the medulla oblongata, also called simply the medulla, with the pons and the midbrain area above. The brain stem performs critical yet basic life-promoting functions, most of which are automatic and ongoing and generally outside of conscious awareness, such as regulation of heart rate, respirations, blood pressure, and scanning movements of the eye. Other mostly automatic activities initiated in the brain stem include swallowing, coughing, and sneezing. In moments of imminent danger, or with internal physiological disturbance, the brain stem response could include fainting or loss of consciousness, or autonomic responses of change in blood pressure and heart rate. The brain stem plays a role in the circadian rhythm within the body, adjusting to a 24-hour cycle of waking and sleeping. With trauma, depression, and accompanying anxiety, there is often disruption in sleep cycles, prevention of restorative sleep processes, and prevention of the brain processing trauma experiences and memories. Assisting and educating clients around the need for reestablishing normal sleep–wake cycles may be a very necessary and important consideration for therapists working with a trauma focus. Chapter 9 will provide the counselor with further information on the neuroscience of sleep and implications for the treatment of trauma.

Sitting at the top of the brain stem is the thalamus. Some consider the thalamus to be part of the brain stem while other sources point out its location in proximity to midbrain structures such as the limbic system. Appropriately, the thalamus is functionally similar to a preprocessing or switch center, relaying messages mostly received from sensory organs or from the brain stem up to cortical areas for interpretation and signal to action. Messages from every sensory organ, except for the olfactory sense of smell, are processed through the thalamus. The thalamus is a critical link for control and regulation of the motor systems located in the brain that influence voluntary movements and general coordination of the body. The thalamus also influences the complexities of the sleep–wake cycle through influence of the pineal gland and the secretion of melatonin.

In the rear portion of the brain at the back of the head is the occipital lobe with the extensive visual cortex, the cerebellum with command of movement and balance, and with the brain stem located underneath. This brain alignment mirrors the evolutionary changes that have occurred over time from reptilian, to mammalian, and upward to the higher level reasoning and functioning centers of the human cerebral cortex. Ever alert for danger, the midbrain constantly scans for confirming information from the five senses. The brain takes a bottom-to-top approach to danger detection and response, with a complex release of neurochemicals and hormones to energize the body to escape the danger. The higher reasoning areas of the brain begin to temporarily disengage, and the midbrain limbic system (including areas that access past memories) responds on high alert. In moments of imminent danger or death, and with no possibility of outrunning or fighting the threat, limbic system functioning halts and the person or animal may, through autonomic nervous system functions, may experience a loss of consciousness or dissociation. Still, the most basic functioning of the brain stem remains intact, and the person continues with the heartbeat and breathing fundamental to survival. As a parallel of sorts, modern medical and surgical procedures, such as the administration of anesthesia, may capitalize on this, allowing consciousness to wane, parts of the midbrain to quiet, and even temporary suspension of usual breathing and brain stem functioning, which is augmented with artificial ventilation. Trauma-aware therapists should be aware of possible post-traumatic effects of surgical and other medical treatment procedures in the history of their clients, particularly in children. On rare occasion, individuals may even report incomplete surgical sedation and can suffer from associated traumatic memories and stress related to these procedures (Osterman et al., 2001).

Concept of the Triune Brain

In the late 1960s, researcher Paul MacLean developed a conceptual model around the organization of the human brain, which included a comparison to other animals' neural system organization and which postulates on the evolutionary course of brain development.

MacLean, in his 1990s book *The Triune Brain in Evolution*, posited a vertical organization of brain consisting of three areas stacked one upon the other. Referring to this as the 'triune brain,' he outlined three layers of the human brain, organizing them according to their appearance in evolutionary development. At the base of the brain, known variously as the medulla or brain stem, is the area of autonomic functioning common to all vertebral animals. The brain stem includes the medulla, the pons, and thalamus, and is connected at the base to the spinal column. Also considered part of the brain stem is the cerebellum, which appears separately like a mini brain at the lower region in the back of the head.

As previously mentioned, autonomic functions such as breathing, heartbeat, temperature regulation, waking and sleeping, basic movement, and a switchboard for receiving circuits for sensory input all have their origin in the brain stem. Referred to as the 'reptilian brain,' this area functions automatically to sustain life. Thus, even following loss of consciousness or higher brain functioning, the brain stem works continually to reestablish homeostasis and proper functioning. To borrow an analogy from the computer world, the brain begins to 'reboot' following injury. The body and the brain begin to come back online slowly, beginning with the lower brain functions and continuing to the higher cortical brain. Trauma therapists will benefit from a basic understanding of this bottom-to-top physiological return to functioning, particularly if working in acute disaster and emergency response settings. It is important in emergency response work for responders to be a calming presence as they assist those who are traumatized. A bottom-to-top awareness of brain functioning would guide therapists to carefully assist clients in the immediate aftermath of trauma. Establishing a safe place with minimal sensory stimulation allows clients to reestablish homeostasis at their own natural pace. Being aware of possible external sensory stimuli is important. For example, the sense of hearing may be intact even though a person is seemingly not conscious or aware. While mental health therapists are usually not present in the immediate moments following severe accidents, health care providers or emergency responders can best serve accident victims by speaking calmly and soothingly and by protecting the victim from bystanders' comments of alarm or doom, as the person may be able, on some level, to hear comments made.

Toward the back lower area of the head is the cerebellum; its shape resembles the cortex in some ways, including having two side-by-side areas similar to each other, in the right and left hemispheres. The cerebellum has a some-what gnarly surface with smaller folds than those of the cortex. The cerebellum has long been thought to be primarily responsible for balance, posture, and proprioception (location of body in space). New research has discovered that the cerebellum has many more functional roles than previously thought. There is indication that the cerebellum may be involved in some level of cognitive functioning, particularly when protective reflexive movement is called for. The cerebellum of an animal such as a cat, known for agility and landing on its feet, is noted to be a proportionately larger than in other animals. Recent research attention has focused on neural pathways leading from the cerebellum to cortical areas of the brain, suggesting that a fresh look at cerebellar functioning may be in order. This research suggests the cerebellum may provide information up to the hippocampus and play a role in sifting through usual incoming sensory information and selecting the novel or unique information to hippocampal memory centers for consolidation (Watson, 2015). The next brain layer is the midbrain, referred to as the Paleo-mammalian brain, which contains the limbic system. This portion of the brain is believed to have evolved with the earliest mammals. The limbic system is involved in behaviors considered more instinctual in nature and is the originator of emotions (see Figure 2.5). It is involved with sexual impulses, anger, and basic survival. Knowledge and understanding of limbic system functioning is critical for therapists, particularly those working with trauma.

The limbic system is made up of a number of parts, all with various functions. There is the hypothalamus, which provides a direct link between the nervous system and the hormonal or endocrine system, chiefly by interaction with the pituitary gland. The hypothalamus is chiefly responsible for the survival protective fight-or-flight response, as it

LIMBIC SYSTEM STRUCTURES

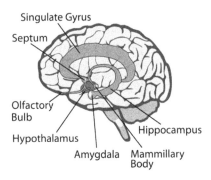

Figure 2.5 Limbic System

initiates a cavalcade of hormonal activation that mobilizes the energy necessary to respond to imminent threat or danger. Then there is the hippocampus, oddly derived from the Latin word for seahorse. The hippocampus is involved in memory formation and spatial awareness. The hippocampus helps to filter fleeting sensory information and to determine whether to send information to long-term memory for consolidation. The hippocampus is part of the limbic system in which memories can get 'stuck' or incompletely processed, resulting in conditions such as PTSD. The limbic system includes the amygdala, whose name refers to the side-by-side almond-shaped structures deep in the brain. The amygdala is primarily responsible for emotional responses, as well as being involved in emotional connections to memories. The amygdala facilitates the nurturing of young, and the conditioned responses to fear. The amygdala receives stimuli from all sensory organs, has a direct link to the olfactory nerve, and is involved with the immediacy of the sense of smell. The olfactory sense is said to be the most primitive and directly connected to the outside environment. Smell information is often processed in the brain before conscious awareness. In Chapter 3 we will discuss the powerful sensory role of olfaction and point to education about treatment adjuncts such as aromatherapy and therapeutic use of scent in mental health treatment.

The brain area sitting above the organs of the limbic system and below the cerebral cortex is known as the limbic lobe. This area is surrounded by the cerebral cortex and therefore sits in contact with the cortex, including areas of the parietal, temporal, and frontal lobes. Contained here is the cingulate gyrus and parahippocampal gyrus. The cingulate functions as bridge or a switch station between the limbic system and the cerebral cortex. The cingulate is thought to have involvement in the unpleasant ruminations and compulsions common in obsessive-compulsive disorder. According to research, neurons extending from the anterior cingulate gyrus to and from the orbital frontal cortex seem to become locked in patterns of over activity "generating the persistent sense that something is amiss" (Schwartz & Begley, 2002, p. 63).

The crowning glory of the nervous system, causing the evolutionary development from which humans became dominant among Earth's creatures in planning, predicting, and problem solving, is the cerebral cortex. This top-sitting part of the brain completes the MacLean triune descriptive model. Again, while being a model that is somewhat simplistic in nature, this top-down and bottom-to-top model provided a conceptual description for a basic introduction to the complexity of the human brain.

Prefrontal Cortex

The dorsolateral prefrontal cortex (DLPFC) is an area of the cortex that sits near the top and side of the brain on both right and left hemispheres. Generally, the cortex area of the brain was thought to be the seat of human uniqueness within the animal kingdom. It was considered to have developed late in terms of evolutionary development and to be present exclusively in primates. Recent research in developmental and comparative neuroscience has pointed out that our uniqueness may not lie in our possession of a prefrontal cortex per se, but to the intricate connections between cortical areas and on throughout the brain (Kaufman, 2013).

Functionally, this area of the cortex, along with the ventrolateral prefrontal cortex, has direct communication with and connection to many different brain areas. These may include connections to the anterior and posterior cingulate gyrus, the striatum, the switchboard-like thalamus, the motor cortex, and the hippocampus. These connections have a strong impact on higher level (also called executive level) functioning of the brain. Specifically, this area is heavily involved in duties of working memory, focused attention, reward and behavioral motivation, and the ability to assess or adapt behavioral responses as required in changing situations (this is also known as 'set-shifting'). The DLPFC helps to determine the important contextual requirements to notice in order to perform a task. In simple terms this is sometimes referred to as the *how* system.

The underside or ventral area of the prefrontal cortex is known as the ventrolateral prefrontal cortex (VLPFC). Similar to the DLPFC, the VLPFC has corresponding right–left hemispheric areas. The right side of the VLPFC is thought to help to determine which information or stimuli requires attendance and to weed out and disregard irrelevant stimuli. This is sometimes referred to simply as the *what* system. The left VLPFC area acts to control and focus attention. This helps in determining which environmental stimuli are most worthy of notice and is tied to working memory. The brain tends to focus attention on novel or exceptional stimuli detected by sensory organs. The brain may actively maintain focused attention and block irrelevant sensory input. At the same time, it reviews working memory to determine precedence, and move to a decision as to whether a response may be necessary. The VLPFC appears to be involved in the ability to choose to delay action and perhaps to resist temptation. Activity in this area of the brain may have implications for understanding the complexity of addiction and risk-taking behaviors.

The right VLPFC is strongly involved in maintaining a state of vigilance and monitoring the environment for potential dangers. Constant states of vigilance may manifest clinically as heightened levels of anxiety and generalized anxiety disorder. Clinically, anxiety and depression are often noted to be co-occurring conditions. Through the technology of neuroimaging, activated areas of the brain can highlight brain activity as it occurs in states of anxiety and of depression. While activity in the right VLPFC appears associated with anxiety, left VLPFC activity seems connected with the ruminating thoughts, focused attention, and problem fixation common in depression. Thus, a depressed individual may be intensely problem focused, may be prone to rumination, and may have difficulty shifting attention to competing stimuli. This is giving rise to hypothesis that depression could possibly be based on an adaptation of the brain, one toward increased consideration and analysis of complex problems, resolutions, or the integration of competing stimuli (Andrews & Thompson, 2009).

Interestingly studies of individuals with damage to these inhibitory areas of the brain may have compensatory increases in creativity and expression arising from other areas of the brain.

Anterior and Posterior Cingulate Gyrus

An important connecting point of functionality between cognition and emotions may lie within the anterior and posterior cingulate cortex. Located beneath the upper cortical area and above limbic system is the cingulate cortex. While the anterior and posterior cingulate are discussed as one area together in a specific inner area of the brain, the anterior cingulate lies toward the front of the head and the posterior cingulate toward the back. The anterior portion is sometimes described as a collar-like area sitting atop the corpus callosum. The anterior and posterior areas appear to differ in function as well. When areas in the anterior cingulate appear active on neuroimaging, there seems an association with affect and emotional expressions. Expressions of behaviors such as empathy, awareness of social cues, and sympathetic reactions when observing pain responses in others are noted here. The anterior cingulate is one brain area active in the brain of the therapist when attuned to the experience(s) related by the client.

The posterior cingulate cortex lies behind the anterior cingulate. While it appears to be related to cognition and to maintaining focused attention, considerably less is known about the actual functions of the posterior cingulate of the brain when compared to the anterior cingulate. It may be involved in internal and external awareness, on focused levels of attention, and in daydreaming and retrieval of autobiographical memories. Through the activation of the posterior cingulate by use of narrative and autobiographical recollections, other integrative brain regions may also be active (Leech & Sharp, 2014).

Insula

Located deep within the brain is an area called the insula or insular cortex. Until recently, this area of the brain has been often overlooked as a subject for study. Recently, neuroscientist Antonio Damasio (1999) noted that the insular cortex seemed involved in establishing somatic markers for emotional states. Damasio developed a hypothesis around 'embodied cognition' that emphasizes body connections with emotion and the continuing influence on cognition and decision making. The theory proposes that conscious thought is continually informed by a visceral monitoring of internal emotional state of the body. Many new directions in clinical treatment of trauma such as somatic based modalities are shifting toward an integration of somatic and cognitive therapies. Other findings that investigate the functional role of the insular cortex are believed to include interpretation of the experience of pain and the pain response. The insular cortex also seems to play a role in the cravings of addiction. A positive, life-enriching action of the insula involves the ability to appreciate and attach an emotional component to listening to music. Future integrative neuroscience approaches to trauma treatment may include activation of insular areas of the brain through music or dance therapies, or may include quieting insular activation in treatment of pain syndromes.

Striatum

Sitting just underneath the cortex lays the brain region known as the striatum. The striatum is located in an area of the brain known as the basal ganglia. The term 'basal ganglia' describes an area of the intersection of many combined neurons, particularly ones involved in voluntary movements. These neurons may act with influence on voluntary movement in either an inhibitory or excitatory manner. Nerve degeneration in this area of the brain results in the tremors and slow halting movements seen in Parkinson's disease. Located within the striatum are structures that include the caudate and the putamen. These two are described together with the term 'striated.' Striatum is based on a Latin word loosely translated as 'striped.' Upon examination, the striatum appears as bands of gray matter layered with white matter; thus its name. Of special note in the understanding of trauma, attachment, and social interaction, the caudate appears to be active in social behaviors and reward system. According to research of Baez-Mendoza and Schultz (2013), the striatum helps integrate incoming social information into coding of social actions and rewards.

Right–Left Lateralization

Another model for understanding the workings of the brain was developed in the 1960s by Roger W. Sperry, who later went on to receive the Nobel Prize in 1981. Sperry, while researching the effects of epilepsy in the brain, discovered that if the corpus callosum were cut and the two hemisphere of the brain were separated, epileptic seizures decreased or were eliminated. Sperry also noted that when neuronal pathways were disconnected, patients developed other curious symptoms such as an inability to name objects that were processed in the right side of the brain, yet they retained the ability to name objects processed in left side of the brain. This led Sperry to suggest that language was controlled by the left side of the brain. Sperry drew upon the much earlier discovery by Pierre Paul Broca, who in 1861 observed a patient who had an inability to articulate words. This patient suffered from what is now referred to as aphasia. At autopsy, this patient was found to have a lesion in the left frontal cortex area of the brain. Broca concluded that the ability to speak resides in the left hemisphere of the brain. Neuroscience has now discovered capacity for language is found in Broca's area of the brain and also in Wernicke's area, both located in the left hemisphere of the brains in 95% of people. Neuroscience researchers have studied language lateralization in association with right- or left-handedness. This is significant because about 90% of people are right-handed. Among left-handed people close to 70% also have language dominance in the left side of the brain. However, in about 30% of left-handed people, language functions are performed using both hemispheres equally (Carter, 2014). Broca's area is involved with planning of speech and activation of the motor vocal apparatus, and is located in the left frontal cortex. Wernicke's area is

involved in understanding and comprehension of language, and is located near the auditory cortex, usually in
the left temporal lobe. While right brain–left brain mapping of functioning can be helpful in understanding brain
functioning, this model is far too simplistic to explain the
complexity and functioning of the human brain. Nevertheless, the differential functioning of right and left brain
hemispheres caught on among popular culture.

There are questions regarding why there is lateralization within the brain, and these questions are centered
on evolutionary purpose. Attempts to determine why the
brain evolved with hemispheric specification rather than
hemispheric redundancy (having duplicate hemispheres
perform in a manner of passing a baton back and forth)
has occupied research. Researchers from Harvard Medical School have made recent discoveries from work identifying 112 different regions of the brain from heathy
volunteers. They discovered that there are more symmet-
ric areas of brain located in the back of the brain than in
the front portions of the brain. This makes sense when one
considers the need for convergence in visual field and the
path of the optic nerve leading from each eye as it crosses
the optic chiasm and travels to the occipital lobe at the
back of the head. Front areas of the brain, specifically the
frontal and prefrontal cortex, are tasked with processing
streams of thought into future planning, problem solving
and abstract reasoning (Zimmer, 2009). Current research
findings have challenged the simplistic notions of various
functions being located exclusively in one or the other hemisphere, and instead points again to remarkable complexity
and resiliency of the brain and nervous system. When the
brain has sustained trauma, either external or internal and
systemic, it has a remarkable ability to find new pathways
and connections and resume varying levels of functioning.

While the degree of recovery can depend on many factors, including age of the person, area of injury, amount of
time between injury and medical assistance, and rehabili-
tation efforts, recovery of function is possible to a degree
never before recognized. This has important implications
for many different clinical areas such as stroke recovery,
traumatic brain injury, accumulated effects of childhood
traumatic experiences, and more. Lateralization of brain
functioning is key to some therapeutic techniques such
as use of mirrors to help alleviate the phenomenon of
phantom limb pain as suffered by amputees, or of physical therapy exercises to help stroke patients regain the use
of opposite-sided movements. There are even case studies
showing promise for helping patients to access the more
emotion-oriented right side of the brain after lifetime patterns of left brain dominance (Siegel, 2010). In her book
My Stroke of Insight, neuroanatomist Jill Bolte Taylor shared
her personal journey when, at age 37, she survived a mas-
sive brain hemorrhage (stroke), which extensively damaged her left hemisphere of her brain (Taylor, 2006). As a
neuroscientist, she was able to observe and later describe
her experience with brain injury as though an outside
observer, watching as her skills of reasoning, language, and
recall slowly slipped away and the right brain inflection
of calm, peaceful magnanimity emerged. Her description
highlights with clarity the effects and surprising results of
hemispheric functioning.

Studies of small children who have undergone hemi-
spherectomy, or the removal of one hemisphere of the
brain, due to life-threatening epileptic seizures, have shown
these children often have remarkable recoveries from this
drastic surgery, some with the only residual effects remaining after surgery of slight fine motor difficulties.

In general terms, there are different but related descriptions of right brain versus left brain functionality (see

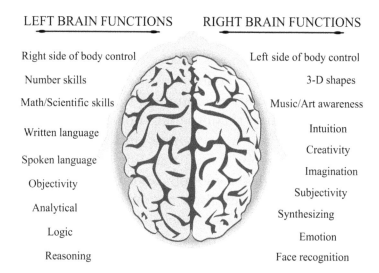

LEFT BRAIN FUNCTIONS   RIGHT BRAIN FUNCTIONS

Right side of body control   Left side of body control

Number skills   3-D shapes

Math/Scientific skills   Music/Art awareness

Written language   Intuition

Spoken language   Creativity

Objectivity   Imagination

Analytical   Subjectivity

Logic   Synthesizing

Reasoning   Emotion

                                                   Face recognition

Figure 2.6 Right–Left Brain Lateralization

Figure 2.6). The left brain is logical, time oriented, goal fulfilling, and talkative. The right brain is observant, connective, and tied into emotions and the bodily experience of emotions. The right brain is holistic and intuitive. It excels at face recognition; in fact, most people can actually better recognize a face if they look at the face with their left eye only (allowing for direct access to facial recognition areas in the right brain). In Western culture, the emphasis on left brain functions dovetails well with the zeitgeist of the people. The drive, energy, and competitive goal-focused behaviors fit well with left brain dominance. Other cultures may have more affinity to right brain functions, such as Eastern cultures, which promote introspection, attachment, and unity.

The following is an example that highlights a counselor's knowledge of brain functioning along with counselor self-awareness and intuition, put to use during clinical assessment and intervention.

Case Example

A brain-wise therapist was perplexed by the couple sitting in front of her. Following a standard assessment and establishing marital counseling treatment goals set by the couple, marital counseling proceeded. However, despite counseling interventions and tool box techniques, the therapist sensed that this couple was simply going through the motions and not fully engaged in counseling. Beneath their notable congeniality and courteous interactions was a deep chasm between them that the therapist couldn't quite pinpoint. Unable to resolve this vague sense or nagging intuition, the therapist took extra quiet, mindful moments of reflection prior to meeting the couple, in order to center herself in preparation for upcoming session. She sat quietly, focused on her breath, and began alternate nostril breathing by specifically and deliberately closing her right nostril and inhaling through her left nostril. She did this in the hope that she might better discern what was going on with this couple. This ancient yoga technique has been said to help quiet the analytical left brain and allow the right brain, with its holistic, intuitive sense, to assist in understanding and perceiving beyond language. The therapist then walked slowly into session, prepared to share with the couple her professional perplexity at their interactions, even to admitting difficulty knowing how to best assist, yet sharing this intuitive sense that she was missing something. The wife arrived to session before her husband. She quietly told the therapist that she had something she wanted to share with the therapist. She began by saying that although she loves her husband, she has long struggled with acknowledging that she is sexually attracted to women and can no longer continue to live with this deception in her marriage. The counselor listened to her client and gave a silent nod within to her intuitive right brain and was able then to shift to the left brain functions of problem analysis, changes in treatment focus, and case conceptualization.

This therapist, in seeking to better understand the complexity of client experience and point of view, used concepts of neuroscience, including right–left hemisphere functioning, in work with clients, particularly in regard to understanding her own nervous system self-regulation. Alternate nostril breathing, also known as unilateral forced nostril breathing, is based on an ancient yoga technique that therapists can use to calm their own autonomic nervous system and heighten their creative, intuitive sense when working with clients. Current neuroscience research of sleep–wake cycles, nasal breathing cycles, and right brain–left brain lateralization may support yoga concepts of the effect of various breathing methods on mind–body and autonomic nervous system functions. The theory is this: The autonomic nervous system influences our sleep–wake cycles, which typically operate in roughly 90-minute cycles throughout a 24-hour day. Interestingly, people tend to also cycle their breathing through one side of the nasal cavity at a time, and then alternate for similar periods throughout the day and night. Physical movements and activities (such as nostril breathing) are controlled by the opposite side hemisphere of the brain. Thus, accessing opposite hemisphere functioning may be aided by temporarily opening breathing to one side for a period of time (Shannahoff-Khalsa, 2001).Therapists can also learn such beneficial breathing techniques for their clinical work, to center and ground before sessions and perhaps gain benefits for their own health and well-being.

Memory and Cognition

Perhaps the most unique and highly studied areas of neuroscience are focused on memory and learning. Fundamentally, memory and learning are based on our awareness of and interaction with the environment, both internal and external. As the brain begins to develop in utero, neurons are connecting and firing together in response to input from the environment. A broad definition of the brain function of memory is "the re-creation of past experiences by the synchronous firing of neurons that were involved in the original experience" (Carter, 2014, p. 156).

While there are many different types of memory, each involving different areas within the brain, they all hold in common their development in response to experience of and interaction with the environment. Experience and exposure are then translated into learning. The learning process occurs on the level of neurons, resulting in actual physical changes in connecting neurons in the brain. Neurons that fire together initially to produce or register a certain experience are altered so they strengthen their connection and increase the likelihood that they will fire together in the future. The complexity of memory is reflected within the variation of human experience. Memory includes everything from learned actions like walking, acquisition of language, and the recitation of facts on an exam, to the instinctual responses to strong stimuli such as a sudden loud noise or a bitter taste.

The recall of memories is impacted by many factors, including whether input is currently held in short-term memory, also known as working memory, which exists to provide us with immediate information and recall, and shortly after this recall is forgotten. Short-term memory allows us to remember the digits of a phone number or verbal directions to a destination. Whether a memory will proceed on to be stored in long-term memory depends on a number of factors, including the emotional content surrounding input, whether it is a new or novel exposure, and whether it is consolidated by rote or repetitive learning exposures.

There are different types of memory, including procedural memory, which allows for the learning of motor actions such as walking or riding a bicycle—actions that once they are learned can be repeated requiring little conscious attention. Procedural memory is active within connections to the cerebellum to assist with coordination and movement, and in the putamen, a part of the basal ganglia, which works to help store in memory a specific learned skill.

Memories can include semantic memory, which stores factual information and simple knowledge, usually without any associated personal context. Semantic memory is encoded in the temporal lobe and accessed in frontal lobe areas for conscious recall.

Working memory may include interpretation and planning based largely upon language areas of the cortex including Broca's area and Wernicke's area.

A type of memory with special relevance to trauma is called episodic memory. Episodic memory includes remembrance of past experiences, including the emotions and physical sensations associated with the experience. This type of memory often includes components of time and place, and plays out with narrative perspective. The specific parts of the brain involved in episodic memory depend in large part on the intensity and content of the original experience. Most episodic memory is initially registered following sensory input, and then processed in the hippocampus where an experience or event may be encoded and consolidated into long-term memory. In the immediacy of a traumatic experience, neurotransmitter and hormonal flooding of the stress hormone noradrenaline sharpens encoding of the sensory aspects of the experience. Sensations of sights, smells, and sounds are all set into memory with vivid clarity. One of the diagnostic criteria for PTSD involves physiological reactivity when there is exposure to external cues that are similar to the encoded memory of a traumatic event. The vivid sensory memory and subsequent physical reactivity places a person in a continuing state of stress. Long-term stress or constant memory triggers also causes the body to release increased cortisol. Chronically elevated cortisol levels have been shown to disrupt hippocampal function (McEwen, 1998). Current research in the trauma field has a focus on memory consolidation, the initial and subsequent fear response and on fear conditioning following trauma. A preliminary research finding indicates that a high level of fear conditioning might be a predictive factor for vulnerability to development of PTSD. Research by Pile et al. (2015) focused on the consolidation window, or the period of time when fearful memory, if blocked, may minimize or prevent future generalized fear responses like the flashbacks characteristic of PTSD. This research highlighted possible preventive aspects of certain psychological therapies administered during the consolidation window following trauma. Further research in trauma points to a similar goal to intervene during the memory consolidation window for possible prevention of PTSD and traumatic memories through the administration of medications such as propranolol to block the effects of the flooding of adrenalin after trauma (Johnson, 2010).

References

Andrews, P.W., & Thompson, A.J. (2009). The bright side of being blue: Depression as an adaptation for analyzing complex problems. *Psychological Review*, 116, 620–654.

Baez-Mendoza, R., & Schultz, W. (2013, December 10). The role of the striatum in social behavior. *Frontiers in Neuroscience*. doi: 10.3389/fnins.2013.00233

Broca, P.P, (1861). Loss of speech, chronic softening and partial destruction of the anterior left lobe of the brain. First published in *Bulletin de la Societe Anthropologique*, 2, 235–238. Trans. Christopher D. Green, 2003. (retrieved March 31,2016 from http://psychclassics.yorku.ca/Broca/perte-e.htm#f1)

Carter, R. (2014). *The human brain book*. New York: DK Publishing revised edition.

Damasio, A. R. (1999). *The feeling of what happens: Body, emotion and the making of consciousness*. New York: Random House.

Gavett, B. E., Stern, R. A., & McKee, A. C. (2011). Chronic traumatic encephalopathy: A potential late effect of sport-related concussive and sub concussive head trauma. *Clinics in Sports Medicine*, 30(1), 179–188, xi. doi: 10.1016/j.csm.2010.09.007

Johnson, K. (2010). Propranolol: A promising treatment for PTSD. *Medscape Multispecialty*, (retrieved August 30, 2015 from www.medscape.com/viewarticle/729444%23vp_2)

Kaufman, S.B. (2013, May 16). Gorillas agree: Human frontal cortex is nothing special. *Scientific American.* (retrieved November 18, 2015 from *blogs.scientificamerican.com*)

LeDoux, J. (2002). *Synaptic self: How our brains become who we are*. New York: Penguin Books.

Leech, R., & Sharp, D.J. (2014). The role of the posterior cingulate cortex in cognition and disease. *Brain*, 137(1), 12–32. http://doi.org/10.1093/brain/awt162

McEwen, B.S. (1998). Protective and damaging effects of stress mediators. *New England Journal of Medicine*, 338, 171–179.

McKee, A.C., & Robinson, M.E. (2014). Military-related traumatic brain injury and neurodegeneration. *Alzheimer's & Dementia*, 10, S242–S253. (retrieved March 31, 2016 from www.sciencedirect.com/science/article/pii/S1552526014001319 doi.10.1016/j.jalz.2014.04.003)

Osterman, J. E., Hopper, J., Heran, W. J., Keane, T. M., & van der Kolk, B. A. (2001). Awareness under anesthesia and the development of posttraumatic stress disorder. *General Hospital Psychiatry*, 23(4), 198–204.

Pile, V., Barnhofer, T., & Wild, J. (2015). Updating versus exposure to prevent consolidation of conditioned fear. *PLoS One*, 10(4), e0122971. doi: 10.1371/journal.pone.0122971

Ratey, J.J. (2001). *A user's guide to the brain: Perception, attention, and the four theaters of the brain*. New York: Random House, Inc.

Schwartz, J.M., & Begley, S. (2002). *The mind & the brain: Neuroplasticity and the power of mental force*. New York: HarperCollins Publishers.

Schwarzbold, M., Diaz, A., Martins, E. T., Rufino, A., Amante, L. N., Thais, M. E., & Walz, R. (2008). Psychiatric disorders and traumatic brain injury. *Neuropsychiatric Disease and Treatment*, 4(4), 797–816.

Shannahoff-Khalsa, D. (2001). Unilateral forced nostril breathing, basic science, clinical trials, and selected advanced techniques. *Subtle Energies Energy Medicine Journal*, 12, 79–106.

Siegel, D. J. (2010). *Mindsight: The new science of personal transformation*. New York: Random House.

Stiles, J., & Jernigan, T.L. (2010). The basics of brain development. *Neuropsychology Review*, 20(4), 327–348.

Taylor, J.B. (2006). *My stroke of insight: A brain scientist's personal journey*. New York: Penguin Group.

Thompson, D. (2014, September 30). Head injuries may raise chances of risky behaviors by teens. *HealthDay*. (retrieved August 15, 2015 from http://consumer.healthday.com/kids-health-information-23/kids-and-alcohol-health-news-11/head-injuries-may-raise-chances-of-risky-behavior-by-teens-692229.html)

Watson, T.C. (2015). "And the little brain said to the big brain . . . "Editorial: Distributed networks: New outlooks on cerebellar function. *Frontiers in Systems Neuroscience*, doi: 10.3389/fnsys.2015.00078 (retrieved June 1, 2015 from journal.frontiersin.org)

Zimmer, C. (2009, May). The big similarities and quirky differences between our left and right brains. *Discover Magazine*.

3

CONNECTIONS

The unique functioning of the nervous system has everything to do with connections. Unlike stand-alone functioning of other organs of the body, the nervous system itself is all about community and networks. Compared to, say, a smooth muscle cell of the heart whose singular purpose is to contract and rest without interruption, a neuron must join up with its neighbors and carry messages and commands throughout the nervous system and body. This networking and communication occurs when neurons in close proximity send their message one to another. This cell-to-cell connection requires close proximity, with only the tiniest of spaces between neurons. This space is called the synaptic cleft or, simply, the synapse. Messages or signals pass in one direction along a dendrite, or axon, carried along by electrically charged ions. The neuron is encased in a cell membrane wall that contains minute channels through which electrical ions may pass. The neuron membrane also has the ability to actively pump electrically charged ions back and forth across the membrane wall. These chemical ions have a positive charge and include sodium and potassium ions. The electrical charge between the fluid inside the cell and the positive ions compels the neuron membrane to pump positive sodium ions into the cell, a process known as depolarization. This process then makes the inside of the cell more positively charged than the outside of the cell, leading the ions in the downstream region of the neuron membrane to move back across the cell wall to the outside area of the cell. This is known as repolarization. When the impulse reaches the synapse, a different chemical reaction takes place at this connection point. The actual space or distance between adjacent neurons at the synapse is miniscule. This allows chemical communication from neuron to neuron to occur by a process of diffusion. Diffusion allows substances to move easily from an area of higher concentration to one of lower concentration. This chemical reaction is mediated by the presence of different chemical substances called neurotransmitters. The resulting chemical reaction causes either an uptake of the signal to the neighboring cell, or an inhibition of the cell signal, depending on a variety of factors.

Focusing on a single individual neuron and its connection to a neighboring neuron would only take us a limited distance in understanding the complexity and functioning possibilities of the brain and nervous system. In considering connection, researchers are now focusing on groups, or networks, of functioning neurons and on the ways they assemble into these groups. These groupings of neurons are known as connectomes (see Figure 3.1). In 2009, the Human Connectome Project began with the intention of mapping the neural connections bundled within the human brain. (www.humanconnectomeproject.org). A goal of the Human Connectome Project is to diagram the wiring and connections of an entire living human brain. This work is being completed by utilizing an advanced MRI technology called diffusion MRI. An example of some new research findings of the Connectome Project have illustrated that groups of interconnected neurons seem to be laid out in a grid-like pattern rather than as a jumbled, tangled pattern of connections as was previously thought (Yong, 2012). Research revelations from this project continue to point to

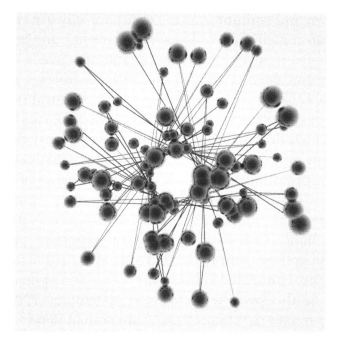

Figure 3.1 Conceptual Model of Connectome

the complexity and intricacy of neurons and connectomes in the brain. It has been said that there are more synaptic connections in the brain than there are galaxies in the known universe.

In addition to neurons and their myriad connections with each other, there are cells called glial cells that serve as a sort of scaffolding, giving physical support to the connecting network of neurons. Types of glial cells called oligodendrocytes (in the brain) and Schwann cells (in the peripheral nervous system) produce an insulation-like covering around the neuron known as a myelin sheath. Much like the rubber or plastic covering around conducting wire, the myelin sheath allows the nerve impulse to travel along the length of the neuron quickly and, within tiny gaps in the myelin sheath, allows for exchange of charged potassium and sodium ions necessary for electric conduction. Star-shaped glial cells called astrocytes are believed to influence neuronal functioning and also play a role in memory and sleep (Purves et al., 2001). Astrocytes are the most numerous type of cells found in the central nervous system, or CNS. New research has expanded the role of glial cells to include providing assistance in electrical conduction from neuron to neuron, in cellular breakdown processes involved in trauma such as occurs in cases of stroke and head injury, and even in the inflammatory processes of degenerative brain diseases such as Alzheimer's disease.

This chapter will further highlight important parts of and connections within the nervous system that extend to neurons connected outside the brain and spinal cord. Known as the peripheral nervous system, or PNS, this includes nerves that branch out from cranial nerves within the brain and from the spinal nerves extending down the spinal column. These branches form a network of nerves that reach throughout the body. The PNS includes three groups according to function. There is an afferent group, which relays messages from body to brain; an efferent group, sending messages from brain to body; and the autonomic nervous system, which works to help regulate the automatic and ongoing maintenance functions of the body. Meanwhile, the central nervous system provides continuing coordination of functioning throughout the nervous system.

Included in the PNS are connections to sensory organs such as the eyes and ears, the 12 cranial nerves, and the autonomic nerves. The CNS provides connection from the PNS to internal organs, skin, and limbs of the body. A neuron that connects to the periphery of the body must be able to transmit a signal down the length of its axon toward its connection point. The peripheral nervous system contains some of the longest single cells in the body. Some neural cells are up to a meter in length. The sciatic nerve, which runs from the base area of the spinal cord to the toes, is thought to contain these longest of human neural cells ("Axon," n.d.). In order for the electrical impulse to progress over the length of the cell, it is necessary to have the coating sheath of myelin, which allows for smooth conduction from point to point. A rough comparison of this is found in the protective plastic coating that runs the length of an electrical cord that allows for a quicker progression of the electrical signal.

There are two different pathways or branches of the nerves within the peripheral nervous system. The afferent branch (known also as the sensory branch) contains neurons that send signals to the brain and includes nerves that detect sensory input from receptor points and relay the message back to the brain with amazing speed. The brain will then interpret the message and may decide to send the information back through the efferent (also known as the motor nerve branch) to the muscles of the body, which spring into action for movement and in active response to the ever-changing environment. At times, the afferent nerves and the efferent nerves may send a signal to each other immediately and directly, in essence with temporary bypass of the cognitive centers of the brain, and shortly thereafter send the signal on to the brain with the ever-slightest delay. This is known as a reflex arc. A common example of reflex arc occurs as a doctor tests patients' patellar (knee) reflex with a quick rubber hammer hit to the knee. Reflex arcs can be essential for survival. Fortunately, we don't always have to stop and wait for analytic interpretations from the cortex; instead, we can jerk our hand away upon contact with a hot stove burner. A sensory (afferent) nerve in the fingertip detects heat, arcs through spinal cord nerves around to a connection with a motor (efferent) nerve, which then signals motion to hand muscles to move away quickly. Only after the protective reflex arc does the signal move to the brain, which then detects the 'ouch' factor and interprets that someone forgot to turn off the burner!

A third part of the peripheral nervous system, the autonomic nervous system, or ANS, includes shared components of the CNS and the PNS. The autonomic nerves control automatic functions in the body involved in heart rate regulation, respiration, and digestion. Also, within the autonomic nervous system are the functions of the sleep–wake cycle, sex, temperature control, and hunger and thirst. The autonomic nervous system connects to glands and body organs that assist the body in maintaining a level of balance. The body has an amazing ability to operate within a stable and consistent range of functioning, to detect and regulate, to spur to action, and to move itself back into balance. This process is called homeostasis. It could be said that a primary nervous system function is to monitor and maintain body balance withstanding a constant barrage of internal and external changes. With every complete breath, our nervous system reflects this fluctuating balance. For example, breathing, while under mostly autonomic nervous system control, maintains an ongoing dance between two branches of the ANS, the sympathetic nervous system and the parasympathetic nervous system. There is slight sympathetic nervous system activation upon inhalation and slight parasympathetic activation when we exhale. Ancient practitioners of yoga realized this and used regulation of breathing as a tool to help calm body and mind. Teaching clients with chronic anxiety and overactivation of the sympathetic nervous system to use their breath to quiet and calm will be further discussed in Chapter 9. Built in to these regulatory functions are feedback detection and feedback loops.

Most functions in the body are aimed toward maintaining balance. When the body or the brain detects an internal change, it will activate mechanisms to reverse the change, bringing it back into balance. For example, brain and body work in connection to maintain a narrow range of body temperature. If the temperature of the blood is too high, it is detected by the neurons in the hypothalamus. The hypothalamus will signal other nerve centers, which send signals to blood vessels in the skin. These blood vessels will dilate and allow heat to radiate off the body. If the temperature in blood is still too high, release of sweat will help to further cool and bring body temperature back into balance.

Homeostasis refers to this tendency of the body to maintain a steady, stable environment. Nerve connections and feedback systems help to regulate a brain–body connection in many ways, including monitoring of organ system functioning and the release of endocrine messengers known as hormones. Usually operating below the level of conscious awareness, the ANS is the ever-steady, constant sentinel keeping us alive, with constant attending to the multitude of internal and external experience.

We are intricately intertwined with the environment around us. This is crucial first for survival as well as for the ability to perceive and experience safety, beauty, and the comfort of social attachment, and to understand our existence both internally and in the world around us. Perception begins with our sensory organs. In this chapter about connections, we will explore the sensory organs that connect and translate the world outside to our body and brain.

The amazing process of nervous system development, including sensory development, begins at conception and results in rapid neuron production and growth, and in the migration of neurons toward connectomes (groupings of similarly functioning neurons) and functioning networks.

The first sensory organ and sensory process to develop and function within the womb is the sense of touch. An infant in utero develops this sense at around 8 weeks of gestation. By 32 weeks of gestation, most every component of the sense of touch is functional, including the perception of temperature, pressure, and pain. Fetal development of other sensory organs, including eyes and ears, begins within 5 weeks of conception with continuing refinement through birth and early childhood. The fetus is able to register and respond by movement to sounds in utero. At birth, an infant has clearest vision only to about 8 to 10 inches, precisely the distance required for gazing into the caregiver's eyes when held and for beginning the visual and interactive dance of attachment and bonding. From the first moments, sensory development and interaction with the environment is critical to life and survival.

As therapists working in trauma, we must consider basic aspects of the sensory experience as being uniquely experienced by each client. This includes the interface of sensory awareness, various methods of treatment, and psychoeducation for clients regarding their own sensory processing techniques for calm, healing, and ANS regulation. We guide clients toward understanding how they typically explore and interact in their world. We provide a safe, calm space for clients to explore the interface between memories, past trauma experience, and impacts on life and current functioning. Beginning with initial client contact, we surround our office space with sensory calming attributes, including soothing colors, sounds, and tactile comforts. We leverage healing through the use of sensory components such as olfactory sense, and we can use auditory and visual calming methods. Chapter 10 will discuss integrative therapy adjuncts using sensory components such as aromatherapy, full-spectrum light exposure for treatment of conditions such as seasonal affective disorder, music therapy, and more.

Case Example

Alexa, a 26-year-old woman, was bright, sensitive, and highly motivated in counseling to relieve past trauma and to develop healthier coping methods than the current quick soothing relief she found in her increasing consumption of alcohol. As is common with trauma, she had great difficulty in telling her trauma story in words. Early in counseling, she spoke of her love of photography and how her camera serves as her 'extra' eyes, as it reflects her feelings and represents her experiences. During her work in therapy, Alexa brought her photographs, her visual experience and representation of her world, in order to explain without using words her inner emotional world. Other clients may choose to incorporate art, music, or poetic language to express their experience of feelings and emotions for which language falls short.

Our eyes contain unique neural cells that are sensitive to light. These nerve cells, called photoreceptors, generate electrical signals as light falls against the back of the eyeball onto the retina. These signals are carried over a right and left optic nerve; they cross over each other in the center area of the brain, and then travel to the occipital lobe at the back of the head and into the visual cortex areas. The visual cortex areas have specialized functions that assist in responding to visual stimuli, passing along information to other brain areas, interpreting the perception of angles, noticing symmetry, color response, response to movement, and to direction. Of extra significance to the trauma-informed counselor is the ventral (underneath) area of visual cortex, which runs along the bottom area of the temporal lobe. This area is connected to memory areas

that enable the recognition of objects according to previous visual memories and exposure. This visual pathway for
facial recognition has evolved, having great importance
to socialization prevalent in the human species. There
appears to be a direct link from the facial recognition area
to the amygdala, resulting in an emotional response to recognized faces. This brain area is developed very early as a
baby begins to cue into the facial expressions of caregivers.
Studies have shown that survivors of early abuse are highly
attuned to minute changes in facial expression (Schore &
Schore, 2007).

In addition to understanding the visual sensory development of facial recognition, the trauma-aware counselor
can review and consider research on visual detection and
the possible physiological effects of color and light. There
has been frequent criticism around lack of efficacy and
evidence-based utilization of light and color in the treatment of mental health conditions, nevertheless, science
is informing us of helpful treatments of exposure to full-
spectrum light sources for conditions such as seasonal
affective disorder. Other effective medical treatments
using light and color are demonstrated by the neonatal
treatment of jaundice using exposure to blue spectrum or
full-spectrum light. As far back as Hippocrates, exposure
to environments filled with light was seen as conducive
to healing (Frumkin, 2003). The trauma therapist can
take care to create a healing environment in counseling
offices to provide soothing colors and lighting. The therapist can teach clients color awareness to aid in developing
a plan for optimal sleep hygiene, including a darkened
room without artificial light from sources such as cellular phones and computers. Color processing begins in the
brain in an area of the visual cortex. Certain color schemes
in counseling offices may be perceived as cold and others
as warm and comfortable or energizing. Colors toward

the red end of the spectrum are often seen as energizing and are reflected within common language, including metaphors for anger (as in, "it made me see red") or sadness ("I'm feeling blue"). An overview of the field called chromo therapy can be found in the review by Azeemi and Raza (2005).

Other therapeutic modalities such as EMDR (Eye Movement Desensitization and Reprocessing) include directed eye movements simultaneous to recollection of traumatic memory. Utilizing bilateral movement of the eyes linked with processing through traumatic memories (or imaginal exposure) is thought to result in a decrease in emotional and physiological distress associated with the memory. Chapter 9 will examine this much touted treatment method in greater depth.

Our ears include neural sensory connections that detect vibrational waves from the environment, travel through the three areas of the ear (the outer, middle, and inner ear), and are converted to electrical signals within the cochlea, a small organ of the inner ear with a unique snail-like shape. This electrical signal then travels along the cochlear nerve, through the thalamus, and on to the auditory cortex, located in the temporal lobe located on the side and lower region of the brain, in close proximity to the ears. The inner ear area also contains the semicircular canals, whose function is akin to a carpenters' level. Fluid inside the semicircular canals responds to positioning of the body and relays vestibular information regarding balance and movement. This function closely interacts with visual sensory input to monitor and assess the position of the body in space, known as proprioception. Sounds received in the ear travel along the auditory nerve to the opposite side auditory cortex, similar to the crossover of the optic nerve with the sense of sight. Perception and interpretation of sound is received first by the thalamus, where sound quality such as intensity, frequency, quality, and meaning are analyzed. There are some hemispheric differences in the perception of sounds, with the left auditory cortex involved in interpretation of meaning and identification of sound, and the right auditory cortex with quality of sound (Carter, 2014).

The brain is able to send signals back to the ears by creating a circuit that can monitor sound input. This gives us the discriminatory ability to focus on a distinct part of a conversation in a noisy room or to block awareness of the running drone of a jet engine during a flight.

The sensory experience of sound through hearing is often a component of developing trauma memories. Recollections of sounds heard in the midst of traumatic experiences are set into memory. The presence of a startle response to auditory stimuli is one of the *DSM-5* criteria for PTSD (American Psychiatric Association, 2013). In fact, a startle response, known as the Acoustic startle reflex, is a normal response to sudden loud sounds in infants in the early months of life. The presence of this startle reflex can be an early indicator of proper and healthy neurological functioning. However, an exaggerated acoustic startle response may occur as a result of traumatic memory and PTSD. An exaggerated startle response is one of the indicators required for diagnosis of PTSD.

At the other end of life, recognition of sound is believed to be one of the last senses to continue just prior to death. Awareness of sound is important for the counselor or practitioner working with acute trauma victims. The calm, human voice can go far in soothing the agitated nervous system, perhaps even a factor in helping to avoid the subsequent PTSD and lock-in of memories of the trauma.

Chapter 9 will highlight some therapeutic ways that sound can be used in treatment modalities for trauma and for wellness and health.

The most primitive and direct connection we have from environment to brain is through our olfactory sense, or sense of smell. Our sense of smell is closely linked to the sense of taste. The mechanism of smell is a chemical one. Located within our nose, special receptors detect airborne molecules from the surrounding environment. The behavior of sniffing brings more air and thus more molecules into the nasal cavity. These molecules bind to receptor sites, which in turn send electrical impulses to the olfactory bulb located in the midbrain right beside the amygdala. At times, the detection of an odor may generate the emotion of fear from the amygdala. The detection of scent is further processed in the olfactory cortex. The sense of smell is unique, with a direct connection into the brain with no filter between, from the outside environment to the inner part of the brain.

The emotion of fear as generated by detection of scent can be protective for survival by informing of the need to escape from danger. Our sense of smell may also lead us, beneath conscious awareness, to attraction to a potential mate or, for newborns, to detecting the presence of mother or caregiver. Scent, when paired with associated memories, can be powerful triggers that lie often just below the level of awareness (Butje et al., 2008). The field of aromatherapy is receiving research attention to determine ways in which smell might be used as adjunct or complementary element in therapy for calming and soothing an activated limbic system. The next case example describes the use of scent in a research-informed manner as autonomic nervous system functioning returns to homeostasis following surgery.

Case Example

Recovery room nurse Sandy has been assigned the care of a 52-year-old gentleman following heart surgery. At bedside, she checks his level of consciousness as his brain progressively comes online as anesthesia gradually wears off. She notices he seems mildly agitated, and his vital signs indicate possible pain response. As an adjunct to pain medications and other postsurgical comfort measures, the nurse places a cotton ball saturated with several drops of pure lavender essential oil at bedside to assist in providing a soothing, healing environment during immediate surgical recovery. The nurse gently verbally instructs the patient to take several deep breaths. With continued monitoring, the nurse notices the patient has quieted, appears less restless, and is increasingly responsive to verbal cues.

Chapter 9 will take an in-depth look at aromatherapy and the sensory use of smell as a tool to help clients calm an overactive sympathetic branch of the nervous system.

The sensory connection for touch is perhaps the most immediate connection from the environment to neural receptors found in the skin. In fact, the skin can be said to be the largest sensory organ of all, with 2,500 associated nerve endings found per centimeter of skin on the fingertips alone. A rough illustration of the brain areas devoted to sensory nerve endings throughout the body, this area known as the primary somatosensory cortex, can be found in the diagram of the homunculus in Figure 3.2.

The homunculus figure illustrates graphically the number of sensory neurons concentrated in various areas of the body and the relative importance of these bodily regions for touch reception. There are numerous types of touch

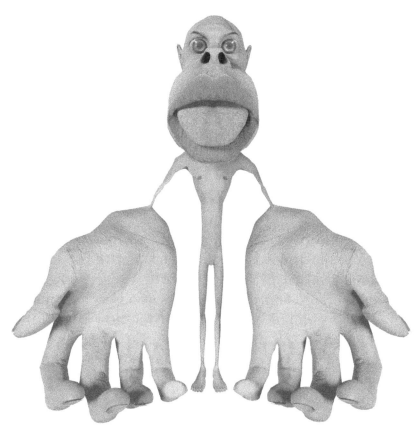

Figure 3.2 Homunculus

receptors that respond to various kinds of environmental stimuli. Different neural receptors can discriminate light touch, pressure, vibration, heat and cold, pain, and proprioception (the perception of movement and the location of the body in space). The importance of the sense of touch is often overlooked, but is critical for early development and healthy attachment, and for emotional development early in life. Well-known studies of infants in Romanian orphanages who were not picked up, held, and touched showed failure to thrive and abnormal brain development and often did not survive. Before this, psychological research on primates conducted by Harry Harlow in the 1950s showed that monkey babies preferred to spend most time cuddled with a soft, warm monkey model alone; this was even preferred over a cold wire momma model that also provided a milky meal (Phillips, 2013). Harlow's, work influenced later research by Bowlby (1988) and others on attachment and the importance of the mother–infant bond.

The importance of the sensory experience of touch has continued relevance for mental health and well-being throughout the life span. For clients who have experienced trauma, touch may evoke through associated memories a triggering and ongoing reminder of past traumatic experience. Yet, the absence of touch may deprive clients of a neurobiological factor in healing. The concept of touch between therapist and client contains necessary and important ethical prohibitions, yet psychoeducation around the importance of touch, and encouragement to clients of not neglecting tactile senses in their healing process, is important. Counselors can provide a tactile-stimulating environment for their clients. The counselor should reach out to clients with a firm handshake to provide tactile connection. Counseling offices can include soft pillows; warm, pleasant temperatures; cuddly dolls and figures for young clients; and even a warm compress for weary shoulders. Referrals to trauma-trained certified massage therapists can be soothing for some clients and provide the neurological benefits of increasing release of oxytocin and serotonin. In disaster response, the focus is on assisting clients in meeting fundamental needs for safety and comfort first; as such, the American Red Cross offers psychological first aid with the addition of a warm blanket for those experiencing acute trauma and aftermath.

An important area of nervous system connection is found in what is known as the vagal nerve pathway. The vagus nerve is the 10th cranial nerve and has many functional roles. It is also the longest of the 12 cranial nerves, stretching from the medulla in the brain stem down through the neck and throat, chest, and the abdomen. The vagus nerve plays a role in maintenance of many bodily functions including swallowing, respiration, heartbeat and digestive functioning. The vagus nerve plays a prominent role in the overall functioning of the autonomic nervous system.

The vagal nerve, as part of the autonomic nervous system, provides connection between neural system to endocrine (hormonal) and immune systems to enable basic physiological functioning. The autonomic nervous system was described as having two branches: the previously mentioned sympathetic (fight or flight) branch and the parasympathetic (rest, digest, and rebuild) branch. The parasympathetic works to sustain and maintain ongoing bodily functions, by assuring a steady supply of oxygenated blood though the heart and circulatory system and by allowing for a steady rate of metabolism. The parasympathetic nervous system tends to slow down the organism, maintaining a balance of basic life functions such as breathing, heart rate, and digestion. The sympathetic nervous system activates the animal for movement and to make a quick response to stress or dangers in the environment.

Research by Stephen Porges, PhD, of the University of Illinois, has provided new understanding about functioning of the ANS and the complex role played by the vagus nerve (Porges, 2009). Porges suggests a possible third role or functioning branch of the autonomic nervous system. In the polyvagal theory, Porges outlines concepts of the actions of parts of the vagus nerve. Its more primitive branch, called the dorsal vagal complex, is found in the dorsal motor nucleus of the vagus nerve. The neurons in the dorsal vagal branch contain no myelin covering and are related to the most primitive physiological maintenance functions of animals like reptiles and amphibians. When danger is perceived, the dorsal vagal branch may mediate a sympathetic fight-or-flight response in connection to the danger. Under extreme duress, and coupled with inability escape the threat, a dorsal vagal response may also include immediate parasympathetic activation, lowering heart and respiration rates and causing the animal to freeze or immobilize to preserve inner metabolism and to feign death. There are animal trainers who recognize this response and solicit it as an entertainment factor when working with animals such as alligators (creating a temporary immobilized state in the animal). Personally, I wouldn't choose to count on such a response if I were to work with or study such animals; I would rather rely on my own sympathetic fight-or-flight response and avoid the danger entirely.

According to Porges, there is evidence for another component of the vagus nerve and autonomic nervous system response. This is believed to be the latest to evolve and is found in mammals, particularly primates. Known as the ventral vagal complex, it includes a myelinated area of the front or ventral side of the vagus nerve. Porges refers to this as the 'social nervous' system. A higher tier or level in evolution can be found when one considers the developmental time required for human brain development. Humans are among the mammals with the longest time from birth to maturity. During this time of rapid brain development that is required for long-term survival until reproductive age, it is necessary for the young to possess tools that elicit through interactions with caregivers a care-taking response. Within the social nervous network are tools that encourage bonding between a newborn and her mother, thus increasing chances of survival. The senses are heightened and develop exquisitely to encourage this bonding. The distance vision of a newborn at birth is about 8 to 10 inches, which is the perfect distance to be able to gaze into his mother's eyes when held at birth. Noting the ever-changing expressions on her mother's face is hardwired into the infant's developing memory and brain connections. An infant's hearing is attuned to his mother's tone and voice from earliest prenatal moments. An infant can identify the smell of its mother over other women. The positive interaction between mother and child in turn results in release of pleasurable, bond-promoting neurohormone such as oxytocin, which creates a loop of attachment and promotes a strong connection between mother and child, which in turn helps ensure protective care of the infant and increased chance of survival.

Research is discovering the detrimental effects of the earliest trauma and the setbacks in brain development of disruption in mother–child attachment. The brain and the nervous system provide ongoing connection both with the environment and inside the body. If connection is disrupted, it can hinder functioning and may result in decreased neural volume in areas such as the hippocampus.

References

American Psychiatric Association. (2013). *Diagnostic and statistical manual of mental disorders* (5th ed.). Washington, DC: American Psychiatric Association.

Axon. (n.d.). *Science Daily.* Retrieved March 1, 2015, from www. science daily.com/articles/a/axon.htm

Azeemi, S.T.Y., & Raza, S.M. (2005). A critical analysis of chromo therapy and its scientific evolution. *Evidence- Based Complementary and Alternative Medicine,* 2(4), 481–488. doi: 10.1093/ ecam/neh137

Bowlby, R.J.M. (1988). *A secure base: Parent-child attachment and healthy human development.* New York: Basic Books.

Butje, A., Repede, E., & Shattelle, M. (2008). An overview of clinical aromatherapy for emotional distress. *Journal of Psychosocial Nursing and Mental Health Services,* 46(10), 46–52.

Carter, R. (2014). *The human brain book.* New York: DK Publishing.

Frumkin, H. (2003). Healthy places: Exploring the evidence. *American Journal of Public Health,* September, 93(9), 1451–1456.

Phillips, R. (2013). Skin-to-skin contact supports optimal brain development. *Newborn & Infant Nursing Reviews,* 13(2), 67–72. (retrieved March 25, 2015 from www.medscape.com)

Porges, S.W. (2009). The polyvagal theory: New insights into adaptive reactions of the autonomic nervous system. *Cleveland Clinic Journal of Medicine,* 76(Suppl 2), S86–S90. doi: 10.3949/ ccjm.76.s2.1

Purves, D., Augustine, G.J., Fitzpatrick, D., Katz, L.C., LaMantia, A.-S., McNamara, J.O., & Williams, S.M. (Eds.). (2001). *Neuroscience* (2nd ed.). Sunderland, MA: Sinauer Associates. Neuroglial Cells. (retrieved March 29, 2016 from www.ncbi.nlm.nih.gov/ books/NBK10869)

Schore, J.R., & Schore, A.N. (2007). Modern attachment theory: The central role of affect regulation in development and treatment. Papers by Yellow Brick Leadership, Springer Science + Business Media, LLC. (retrieved March 21, 2015 from @ *yellowbrickprogram.com)*

Yong, F. (2012). The brain is full of Manhattan like grids. *Phenomena: A Science Salon Hosted by National Geographic Magazine,* (retrieved June 3, 2015 from phenomena.nationalgeographic. com)

4

THE COMMUNICATORS

The explanation of how an individual neuron communicates with its neighbor neuron, and on down the line of connecting neurons, involves a complex chain of actions. This actual communication of nerve impulses is known as spikes, or neural firing. The possibility of communication, of whether a neuron will communicate to its neighbor, is known as the action potential. Nerve impulses, or spikes, usually travel from one neuron to another with amazing speed. Depending on the type of neuron and on factors such as the integrity of the myelin sheath covering the axon, an impulse can travel at amazing speeds of up to 100 meters per second. Two processes are at work each time a nerve impulse is communicated from one neuron to another. The neuron-to-neuron communication occurs through both chemical means and electrical conduction. While the nerve impulse is carried from one end of the nerve cell down the length of the cell, communication of the cell to its neighbor happens in the small space in between, known as the synapse. At the end of both a sending neuron and a receiving neuron there is an area aptly named the synaptic cleft. Produced within the main body of the cell are molecules known as neurotransmitters. Neurotransmitters are carried within bubble-like containers called vesicles. These neurotransmitter vesicles are then carried along through the neuron to the synaptic cleft.

At the end of each synaptic cleft there is a membrane through which the tiny vesicles of the neurotransmitters are able to easily pass; the vesicle breaks open and releases the neurotransmitter, which then fits into the same shaped receptor in the adjoining cell. In this manner an impulse may continue onward with a new wave of electrical depolarization of each successive neuron.

There are many different neurotransmitters that enhance or encourage communication from neuron to neuron. These are called excitatory neurotransmitters, as they help to continue the nerve impulse in its onward travel. There are also neurotransmitters that are called inhibitory neurotransmitters, as they may inhibit or prevent the nerve impulse from traveling. This is accomplished primarily by preventing depolarization from taking place. Whether a nerve impulse is activated or inhibited depends on the kind of membrane channel present on the receiving cell. To put it simply, whether a neuron will fire or spike depends on the balance between the excitatory and inhibitory neurotransmitters. For this reason, neurotransmitters are sometimes referred to as modulators. The communication between neurons involves either the release or the taking up of neurotransmitters at the synapse. These are all important factors necessary for carrying forward the action potential (or firing) of one neuron to another. These chemical molecules are crucial to functioning. While there are many different types of neurotransmitters, they can all be chemically related to one of three groups: the amines (or monoamines), which includes dopamine, histamine, serotonin, and norepinephrine; the amino acids such as glutamic acid, aspartic acid, and gamma amino butyric acid (GABA); and the stand-alone group, which contains acetylcholine. The interplay of various neurotransmitters is like a symphony, and the problems that can occur when the symphony is out of balance have prompted the pharmaceutical world to develop chemical treatments that may mimic actions of neurotransmitters. These treatments may work by increasing the availability of amounts of neurotransmitter in the synapse either by flooding the synapse or by preventing the reuptake of neurotransmitter back into the neuron, which also results in increases in the amount of neurotransmitter found in the synapse.

Because of the tendency in Western cultures to prescribe medication for treatment of disorders of brain and body functioning, some neurotransmitter-acting medications have become among the most commonly prescribed medications. Antidepressants and medications for treatment of conditions such as attention deficit disorder are among the most commonly prescribed medications in this country. Meanwhile, new technologies of brain imaging are showing the effectiveness of other treatment options, including psychotherapy, in increasing connection and formation of new neural networks and in supporting neural connections (Dichter & Smoski, 2008; Karlsson, 2011). Perhaps these discoveries will result in a shift in focus and renewed consideration of the most effective and beneficial treatments available for behavioral health.

Nevertheless, it is important for the therapist, and the trauma therapist in particular, to understand the basic actions of various neurotransmitters and their dominant effect on neurologic and physiological functioning.

Let's take a first look at some excitatory neurotransmitters:

Acetylcholine—widely distributed throughout the central and peripheral nervous systems, whose actions are involved in muscle contraction and in stimulating the release of various hormones. Within the central nervous system, acetylcholine is involved in wakefulness, attention, anger and aggression, sexual behaviors, and thirst, among other functions. Research on acetylcholine has found that a deficit in acetylcholine can be associated with Alzheimer's disease.

Glutamate—the major excitatory neurotransmitter associated with memory and learning. Deficits in glutamate are also associated with Alzheimer's disease, whose early symptoms include deficits in memory. It is estimated that over half the neurons in the central nervous system have receptors for glutamate, which functions to strengthen the link between neurons. In this manner it is also believed to be strongly involved in consolidation of long-term memory.

Aspartate—chemically similar to glutamate and also fits many neuroreceptors sites in the central nervous system, but the effects seem to be weaker.

Norepinephrine and epinephrine (sometimes called noradrenaline and adrenaline)—norepinephrine functions primarily as an excitatory chemical, and it is produced mostly in an area of the brain called the locus coreuleus. The locus coreuleus is located within the brain stem in the pons. Epinephrine (as it is called when found in the body rather than the brain) functions in the body as a neurohormone, being produced in lesser amounts from the adrenal glands located above the kidneys. Epinephrine is released here into the blood, where it helps in maintaining homeostasis and balance of automatic functioning of the body, particularly within the cardiovascular system. Epinephrine is perhaps best known as the fight-or-flight chemical, which allows for responses of great strength and endurance when confronted with life-threatening danger. This specific neural stress response pathway is identified as the hypothalamic-pituitary-adrenal (HPA) axis. The HPA axis involves signals sent from the hypothalamus to the pituitary gland and on to the adrenal glands, which trigger the release of several stress response hormones. There are many receptor sites within the brain that bind to norepinephrine. In this manner, this excitatory neurotransmitter is spread to different areas of the brain, including the amygdala, eliciting a fear response; the hippocampus, with memory imprinting; the hypothalamus and the thalamus with an activating, pay-attention-now switch that is turned on. An understanding of norepinephrine and the fight-or-flight response is critical for counselors working from a trauma-informed approach. The *DSM-5* diagnosis of acute stress response describes many symptoms that occur following the physiological release of stress hormones like epinephrine. Such *DSM* indicators as noted describe heightened sensory activation and awareness, memory consolidation, and hypervigilance and are often accompanied by fear and avoidance. It is clear that the flooding of the system with excitatory hormones such as noradrenaline allows for immediate action to escape from danger. However, the evolutionary development of this complex response to environmental dangers has not kept up with current requirements of humans to cope with the increased ambient stress and urgency of modern times.

Histamine—functions as an excitatory neurotransmitter in the brain. It also plays a great role in the inflammatory response of the body, which is tied in closely with the immune responses of the body. This explains how antihistamine medications (those that work to block the response of histamine) so commonly used during allergy season to dry up drippy noses also can have a side effect of drowsiness by quieting the excitatory response of histamine in the body.

Let's take a look now at some of the common inhibitory neurotransmitters:

Gamma amino butyric acid—the major inhibitory neurotransmitter located throughout most of the brain and nervous system. It is estimated that 30% to 40% of synapses in the brain are receptive to the action of GABA. The presence of GABA inhibits (or decreases) the action potential of the neuron, thereby decreasing the chance of passing a neural spike on toward neighboring neurons. GABA influences motor control in the body, vision, and other functions. Of importance to the study of trauma, GABA is believed to play a strong role in the regulation of anxiety. Antianxiolytic, or antianxiety drugs such as benzodiazepine, work by allowing increased amounts of neurotransmitter GABA to flip the off switch for nerve cell transmission.

Dopamine—can have either an excitatory or inhibitory affect, and it also functions both as a neurotransmitter and as a neurohormone. It is produced in several areas of the brain, including the midbrain region called the substantia nigra, and is released by the hypothalamus. Dopamine helps to make voluntary movement in the body possible. The presence of dopamine plays a role in reward seeking and motivation. It also has an effect on attention, mood, pleasure-seeking behaviors, and sleep. Dopamine is involved in learning processes and working memory. Deficient amounts of dopamine are part of the etiology of Parkinson's disease and are believed to play a role in addiction. Excess amounts of dopamine have been implicated in schizophrenia.

Serotonin—neurotransmitter of particular importance in behavioral health. Serotonin is involved in many various functions in the body, including regulation of body temperature, sleep, appetite, and perception of pain. It is also the chemical highly related to mood. Imbalances of serotonin are related to depression, suicide, risk taking, and impulsive behaviors and aggression. Popularly prescribed medications for treatment of depression and mood disorders are called SSRIs (selective serotonin reuptake inhibitors), which work at the neural synapse to help prevent the gathering up of serotonin at the synaptic juncture and thus keep the synapse awash with serotonin. Higher levels of serotonin are associated with optimism and serenity.

The trauma-informed therapist should develop working knowledge of functions of neurotransmitters and their relationships to behavioral health conditions. While commonly influenced through pharmaceutical treatments of drugs such as Prozac, Xanax, and many more, the counselor can be instrumental in also helping clients to recognize the importance of good basic health practices that can influence the effectiveness of proper neurotransmitter functioning. Psychoeducation on good dietary practices such as the adequate intake of vitamins and nutrients necessary for production of neurotransmitters is important. This includes vitamins such as vitamin D, which is important for production of the monoamine neurotransmitters such as dopamine, norepinephrine, and serotonin. Vitamin D levels can be assessed by laboratory testing and supplementation encouraged by medical recommendation. The water-soluble B vitamin group, particularly B12, B6, and folate deficiencies, are related to depression. Since the B vitamins are not stored in the body, adequate recommended dietary intake is important to promote good nervous system functioning. Good mental health is also strongly associated with omega oil intake. When working with trauma clients and behavioral health clients, a counselor needs to first assess basic physiological functioning including adequacy of diet, rest and sleep patterns, exercise levels, and overall physical health and functioning. When various mental health treatment modalities are being considered, a counselor should not overlook attention to these basics.

Along with functioning of neurotransmitters, there is an extensive network of neurohormones that have critical importance in physiological functioning of the body. These neurochemicals aren't categorized as either excitatory or inhibitory; rather, they are often referred to as modulators. Several neurohormones are produced in the hypothalamus, sent on to the pituitary gland, which then sends the messages to target glands signaling action. The hypothalamus is considered the link between the nervous system and the endocrine system of the body. One such pathway previously mentioned, the HPA axis, sends signals from the hypothalamus to the pituitary gland, which in turn sends information to target glands in the body through the autonomic nervous system. For example, in the HPA axis, the pituitary gland releases the chemical ACTH (adrenocortical tropic hormone), which signals the adrenal glands to release adrenalin and cortisol throughout the bloodstream and on to target areas in the muscles, the heart, even to the muscles around the pupils of the eye. The hypothalamus also has many ongoing functions that maintain and sustain internal activities such as controlling body temperature, appetite and fluid intake, and regulating the sleep–wake cycle. The proximity to and interaction with the limbic system allows for a critical response to stress, both internal and external to the body.

Some of the neurohormones and their actions include the following:

> *Glucocortisol*—also called cortisol. It is a main player of the neurohormones in relation to stress responses. Cortisol is responsible for influencing activation of

the HPA axis in times of stress. Cortisol has many effects on the body, and works closely with body systems as needed to regulate fat, carbohydrate, and protein metabolism, and to assist in production of glucose necessary for the energy needs of the body. Cortisol helps regulate blood pressure and cardiovascular functioning, and influences the sleep–wake cycle and circadian functions. Cortisol levels normally rise and fall throughout the day in a regular, ongoing fashion. In a healthy individual, the cortisol-like stress response counterpart epinephrine kicks in during times of stress to prepare body and mind for action when danger is detected. In early moments and imminent danger, epinephrine is released; the body is activated, prepared, and ready to take steps required to preserve life and limb. Cortisol, the other stress hormone, is released more slowly and steadily to back up the chances of survival. The cortisol released in acute stress responses will temporarily suppress functions of the body that are reparative in the long term, such as immune functions, and instead provide a burst of energy, increased memory, and a decreased sensitivity to pain. Cortisol is supportive of and allows for actions required for evasion of danger. However, if cortisol levels remain elevated for prolonged periods, the adrenal glands become overworked, resulting in lower levels of release of cortisol, decreased immune system functioning, and the susceptibility to bodily damage from wear and tear. New research in the emerging field of epigenetics shows that chronically low levels of cortisol can be found intergenerationally following extreme trauma and hardship (Yehuda et al., 2011). Epigenetics and trauma implications will be discussed in the final chapter of this book.

Oxytocin—sometimes called the "trust hormone." Oxytocin is garnering attention for its possible protective
and positive effects in moments of environmental
trauma. It is produced in the hypothalamus, stored
in the pituitary gland, and released throughout the
bloodstream to the many sensitive receptor sites
located throughout the body. It is the powerful hormone that leads to contractions of the uterus during
and after the birth process, and promotes the early,
important mother–infant bond. It sustains lactation
functions postpartum. The release of oxytocin is
related to euphoria and pleasure during sex, and perhaps strengthens the bond between sexual partners.
New research has shown that oxytocin influences
memory consolidation by blocking some memory
pathways. It is also known as the "social hormone,"
encouraging social affiliation, and allowing the body
to cope and adapt in emotionally charged or stress-
ful situations. In the aftermath of disaster, and in the
face of traumatic stress, the overwhelming and under-
standable desire of humans is reconnection with loved
ones. The importance of connection and attachment,
and of *re*connection following trauma and distress,
coupled with neuroscience in understanding mechanisms of actions of neurohormones like oxytocin,
show promise for future research and understanding.

An automatic function of the communicators (neurotransmitters and neurohormones) is the function of
feedback and the presence of feedback loops. While neurohormone pathways allow for targeted internal actions,
there must also be a mechanism that can signal back to the
nervous system that the necessary action was completed,
and return to state of homeostasis is now underway. While
return to steady state baseline is intricate and complex, it

must be understood as a model for conceptualizing resilience and trauma treatment. Learning how the body and nervous system return to previous levels of functioning can steer us to new ways to understand and provide effective treatment for conditions like PTSD.

References

Dichter, G.S., & Smoski, M. (2008, September 1). Effects of psychotherapy on brain function. *Psychiatric Times.* (retrieved March 3, 2015 from www. psychiatrictimes.com)

Karlsson, H. (2011, August 11). How psychotherapy changes the brain. *Psychiatric Times.* (retrieved March 29, 2015 from www.psychiatrictimes.com)

Yehuda, R., Karesten, C.K., Galea, S., & Flory, J.D. (2011). The role of genes in defining a molecular biology of PTSD. *Disease Markers,* 30, 67–76. doi: 10.3233/DMA-2011-0794 IOS Press

5

TRAUMA AND THE BRAIN

In order to understand the effects of trauma on the brain, the body, and the nervous system, it is helpful to define what 'trauma' is. In 2014, the Substance Abuse and Mental Health Services Administration (SAMHSA) wrote the following definition:

> Trauma results from an event, series of events, or set of circumstances that is experienced by an individual as physically or emotionally harmful or life threatening and that has lasting effects on the individual's functioning and mental, physical, social, emotional, or spiritual well-being.

This definition is suitable to use as a springboard to understanding trauma on the pared down level of the individual brain. It is helpful here to refer back to Chapter 2 and to MacLean's' concept of the triune brain. The limbic system structures of the brain evolved as a constant guard on the lookout for potential environmental hazards and threats to well-being. The primary way the limbic system detects threats is through interpretation of environmental data input received from the five senses. Previous exposure to trauma may also have resulted in consolidation of memory fragments of the trauma event or exposure. Through an ever-vigilant and watchful limbic system, subtle and now generalized cues for danger may be detected, based on previous memory connections from earlier sensory experiences. Interestingly, some forms of sensory input may be interpreted as dangerous not only on the basis of individual exposure and memory, but seemingly through multigenerational or cultural repetition. For example, young children of many different cultures seem to have similar fear, on visual exposure, to long stick-like objects resembling snakes. An example of an innate auditory cue for fear is the universally unpleasant high-pitched screeching sound like fingernails against a blackboard (with apology to younger readers who may be unfamiliar with blackboards). The hypothesis is that screeching sounds might be connected to generational memory of ancient predators.

When the ever-watchful limbic system receives sensory data of possible danger, a cascade of physiological events may take place, all of which having basic, immediate survival as the desired outcome. The response of the individual in immediate danger may include fight, flight (or running away from), freeze, or even faint. Which response or combination of responses an individual is likely to make depends on many factors, including previous exposure to trauma, whether the individual is restrained and unable to flee, having factors supportive to resilience, and more. Let's take a moment and outline the nervous system involvement in each of these acute responses to traumatic events.

The fight-or-flight response is dominated by sympathetic nervous system activation. When danger is detected, the HPA axis, beginning with the hypothalamus, is stimulated to release regulator chemical messengers called corticotropin releasing factor within central nervous system neurons; this activates the pituitary gland, which then signals the adrenal glands to release a further burst of stress response hormones (Smith & Vale, 2006). This hormone release galvanizes the body to action, affecting the heart with increasing heart rate and increasing blood flow to lungs, brain, and muscles throughout the body. It enables the individual to take quick evasive action or to push away the danger. Stories of mothers having bursts of strength to fight danger threatening their children are common, as are stories of strangers jumping into action to push away or rescue another from life-threatening forces. These are examples of stand-and-fight sympathetic nervous system responses. Equally powerful, but perhaps not as dramatic, are stories of individual attempts and rescuer assistance given to help others escape from danger. There are studies in many fields about individual behavior in moments of imminent disaster, which are helping us to better understand, and hopefully to predict, likely fight-or-flight responses. In some cases, responders, soldiers, and others may receive extensive training to inhibit or augment the inherent physiological tendencies toward the four Fs: fight or flight, freeze or faint. For example, research in the field of disaster response and preparedness has shown first responders and emergency planners how to override personal responses of fear and assist, encourage, and increase compliance with evacuation orders during disasters. Predicting whether people will leave (flight) or will stay with seeming defiance to danger (fight) is important for planning how to better assist individuals and communities during disasters. Emergency planning should include and factor in if possible the tempering and calming effects of attachment and social connection, as neuroscience findings indicate. The importance of locating and assisting loved ones, and assuring safety during disaster, all point to neuroscience principles during disaster regarding social engagement network pathways in the brain. Social behavioral awareness, connections, and informed responses, particularly in time of stress, are a promising yet challenging area for neuroscience research. Turning to others, seeking guidance during disaster, may provide opportunity to demonstrate activities of the calming components of vagal social engagement system. For example, it is well-known that people may refuse to evacuate unless the safety of loved ones, including their pets and animals, can be assured; again, this is the social engagement branch of the autonomic nervous system at work. These are examples of some complex neurological processes involved in the face of perceived environmental threat. Again, fight and/or flight are sympathetic nervous system–induced responses. When the perception is that escape is not possible, or that the fight option is being lost, there may be concurrent activation of the parasympathetic nervous system. This polyvagal response puts the brakes on sympathetic functioning, resulting in a freeze response or even sequential breakdown of neurological functioning, including possible loss of consciousness or fainting. In mammals such as the opossum, this faint response is a default response; the animal freezes, with the survival possibility that a predator will lose interest in the (apparently) dead animal and leave it alone. It is also thought that a parasympathetic response, along with the release of cortisol and other neurohormones, provides a pain-abating response in preparation for death.

The work of trauma researcher and clinician Pat Ogden (2011) provides a model that illustrates various levels of affective functioning and mechanisms of autonomic nervous system regulation. Expanding on the concept of 'window of tolerance' introduced by Siegel (1999), Ogden's work provides deeper understanding of nervous system regulation and suggests therapists can assist clients in learning and experiencing self-regulation of nervous system functioning. In working with trauma-affected clients, it is first necessary to help clients reestablish a balanced state between levels of nervous system hyper or hypo-arousal. Assisting clients to access the physiological experience and sensation of calm is a crucial first step toward later work in processing trauma-related material. The window of tolerance concept can be viewed, perhaps whimsically, as a Goldilocks approach (a nervous system not too activated, not too immobilized, but at a just-right level) of nervous system functioning. Chronic overactive sympathetic nervous system arousal results in anxiety, hypervigilance, and an inability to process information and problem solve within cortical areas of the brain. An underactive or parasympathetic response may result in immobility, numbness, or dissociative responses. This tendency may also appear as the immobility and disconnection common in chronic depression. A goal in treatment of trauma is to help the client bring autonomic nervous system functioning into a healthy fluctuating yet overall state of physiological balance as discussed in Chapter 3. Often, clients come to therapy in a chronic state of hyperarousal. This level of functioning eventually results in wear and tear or breakdown, and can have a negative effect on all areas of functioning. Other clients manage to function in a chronic state of hypo-arousal, with the numbness of depression or even a state of dissociation as found in suboptimal levels of autonomic nervous system functioning. It has been said that an average person with PTSD may have been suffering for up to seven years before seeking mental health assistance. As outlined in Chapter 6, a therapist's early task is to help the client establish a sense of safety, with even the therapist office space itself perceived as comfortable, calming, and safe. Later, the therapist can help the client access the desirable range within the window of tolerance, and learn self-regulation of nervous system response. This goal will be discussed further in the remaining chapters of this book.

References

Ogden, P. (2011). *Affect regulation, attachment and trauma: A sensorimotor approach.* Boulder, CO: Sensorimotor Psychotherapy Institute, Training on March 5, 2011.

Siegel, D. (1999). *The developing mind.* New York: Guilford.

Smith, S. M., & Vale, W. W. (2006). The role of the hypothalamic-pituitary-adrenal axis in neuroendocrine responses to stress. *Dialogues in Clinical Neuroscience, 8*(4), 383–395.

Substance Abuse and Mental Health Services Administration. (2014). *Trauma-informed care in behavioral health services.* Treatment Improvement Protocol (TIP) Series 57. *HHS Publication No.* (SMA) 14–4816. Rockville, MD.

6

THE THERAPIST
IMPERATIVE

It might be said that becoming a trauma-informed therapist is a primary goal at the heart of the mental health profession. Arguably, every client seeking the assistance of a therapist is coping in some way with trauma. Counselors and other behavioral health specialists are tasked with understanding neuroscience, brain–body interactions, and the impacts of environment on the nervous system, all while leveraging a social neurological connection for treatment. In other words, counselors must also have self-awareness of their own neurological processes while interacting with and guiding their clients toward nervous system self-regulation. Even the somewhat related helping professions like coaching, which ostensibly is future focused and emphasizes positive coping and skill development, still seeks to provide people with skills that can be helpful in moments of stress and to assist people in moving beyond old memory scripts and small traumas that keep them stuck.

In times of rapid change, people and the societies in which they live must struggle to adapt to stress and change. In the 1940s, sociologist Emile Durkheim conducted research that attempted to bridge a connection between the personal, seemingly isolated individual behaviors of suicide with environmental sociocultural factors, all during times of great change and transition. Durkheim pointed to the rapid change and displacement of people post–World

War II and found correlation between societal change and elevated suicide rates in countries with the greatest levels of change and transition. While such explorations of social, cultural, and traumatic environmental influences may seem to have little to do with understanding of neuroscience and the brain, a new area of study called epigenesis is highlighting how such environmental factors may play out in the genetic expression and inheritance of an individual. The work of Yehuda and others highlights the possible effects of environmental trauma on genetic expression and the possibility of intergenerational manifestations of trauma genetically handed down through altered gene expressions (Yehuda & Bierer, 2009). The concept of epigenesis will be revisited in Chapter 10 in a brief exploration of this new area of neuroscience research.

Currently societies are grappling with accelerated change in new and fundamental ways including climate change, rapid technological advances, and social fragmentation of families and communities. These changes make it likely that few individuals will escape environmental challenges and the experience of trauma. It is well-known, however, that the majority of people who experience trauma do not go on to develop symptomatology of PTSD. Neuroscience research may begin to focus on the process of adaptation to trauma and effective coping. Therapists working with clients must be trauma informed, but also trained in concepts of neuroplasticity and resilience. The therapeutic focus will include being supportive of the natural tendency toward function and adaptation, and of guiding clients toward resilience. The therapist must become the oft quoted 'amygdala whisperer,' through creating a therapeutic setting of calm and connection, upon which the client can begin to reestablish affective self-regulation.

The trauma- and neuroscience-informed therapist can develop a comprehensive approach to all aspects of therapeutic intervention. From first contact with a client, through screening and assessment, treatment planning, and implementation, the therapist must see the client in front of her through a lens of universality and humanity toward the experience of trauma. The therapist needs to hold belief of acceptance regarding the courage of clients as they take their first tentative steps to heal from trauma. The therapist will establish the therapeutic environment that is both literally and interpersonally conducive to the sense of safety and calm for the client. Establishing rapport and trust is essential within the process, as therapy becomes a safe holding vessel for painful emotions, traumatic memories, and difficult perceptions. The assessment phase of therapy should include assessment and self-report of current physiological functioning, as well as attention to behavioral health indicators for trauma. Intake assessments should include various indicators of physiological functioning, including history of frequent or chronic illness and immune system functioning, history of head injury, history of past surgeries or medical traumas, and trauma history and experience with grief or loss. Intake assessments should also include assessment for possible disruptions in early attachment.

An older traumatic experience assessment tool looked at recent individual traumas and possible effects on general health and well-being. This tool, called the Social Readjustment Rating Scale, applies numeric value to some typical and commonly experienced life traumas that may have occurred over the past year in the life of clients (Holmes & Rahe, 1967). The scores from each section are added together and the results are cumulative, with a higher cumulative score being correlated with increased future risk of negative health effects, stress related illness and accidents. Frequently, clients may not recognize, remember, or associate the impact of various life events with current physical and mental health concerns. For example, prior history of head and neck injuries may not come to mind as related to current nervous system dysregulation. Recent attention to brain injury has been spotlighted in the field of sports and also in education, with protocols developed for proper treatment post injury that allow the brain to heal and recover from trauma. The trauma-informed counselor will keep abreast of such research and treatment recommendations for the best interest of clients.

Case Example

A 33-year-old emergency medical technician came to counseling requesting to learn better management of his anger. He discussed how he felt angry and jealous at his girlfriend's interactions with her ex-spouse. He acknowledged that he had no reason to doubt his girlfriend's commitment to their relationship, but couldn't seem to control his angry verbal outbursts whenever he felt anxious. He mentioned that he hadn't always been so quick to anger. When asked when he first noticed a change toward angry outbursts, he answered he had noticed a change 4 to 5 years ago. Questioned further about life events around this time, he reflected briefly, and then replied that he had been hospitalized following a motorcycle accident. He described the accident as involving extensive broken bones and surgery to the left side of his body. When asked about injury to his head and neck, he said that the severity of his injuries probably included head injury and concussion, but he believed that his helmet had protected him. After lengthy physical recovery, he was left with no visible after effects. He didn't at first make a connection between any current behavioral issues to lingering difficulties as a result of the accident. He explained, "Recovery was hard and long, but I thought I had put it all behind me."

> This client never considered that there might be a connection between his previous physical injury and trauma to his current emotional and relational distress.

This example highlights the importance of trauma-informed assessment and treatment planning. The trauma-informed therapist will combine holistic assessment with knowledge of neuroscience to formulate case conceptualization and treatment planning.

Treatment of trauma is evolving rapidly. Neuroscience findings, an influx of returning military veterans, and responses to large-scale natural and man-made disasters precipitate a new and changing focus for the trauma therapist. The Adverse Childhood Experience (Felitti et al., 1998) data points to the peril of early and ongoing trauma to developing brains and to mind and body connections in the development of chronic disease. The following chapters will examine what it means to heal and recover from trauma and how therapists can provide guidance and support to clients on a healing journey.

References

Felitti, V.J., Anda, R.F., Nordenberg, D., Williamson, D.F., Spitz, A.M., Edwards . . . Marks, J.S. (1998). Relationship of childhood abuse and household dysfunction to many of the leading causes of death in adults. *American Journal of Preventive Medicine*, 14(4), 245–258. http://doi.org/10.1016/S0749–3797 (98)00017–8

Holmes, T.H., & Rahe, T.H. (1967). "The social readjustment rating scale." *Journal of Psychosomatic Research*, 11, 213.

Yehuda, R., & Bierer, L. M. (2009). The relevance of epigenetics to PTSD: Implications for the DSM-V. *Journal of Traumatic Stress*, 22(5), 427–434. doi: 10.1002/jts.20448

7

WHAT DOES IT
MEAN TO HEAL?

Healing of mind and body following trauma is complex. First, how might healing be defined? Descriptions of trauma healing could include individual experience with neurological realignment following trauma, or an exploration of intergenerational links of traumatic experience and possible epigenetic changes seen over time, or even of trauma healing and recovery from an entire societal point of view. All of these areas weave in patterns, intertwined, with one affecting the other. Therapists who assist clients can begin with a framework of resilience, and consider the factors supporting the ability to heal. Therapists can leverage personal resources supportive of resilience, and understand both the commonality and individual differences of brain functioning, particularly after trauma, as they support clients toward trauma recovery.

Bottom-to-Top Healing Process

Bottom-to-top healing refers to early trauma work to calm and stabilize lower brain and midbrain activation following exposure to trauma and to subsequent trauma triggers. Bottom-to-top healing has a goal of quieting states of hyperarousal of the sympathetic nervous system, of promoting stability and reconnection in states of hypo-arousal, and of a rebalancing of functioning of the autonomic nervous system. Moving toward top-brain functions allows for memory consolidation, integration, and increasing the neural connections to cortical processing brain areas. It is about helping clients learn to self-regulate and learn to operate within their individual window of tolerance. A revisit to the classic Maslow's hierarchy of needs dovetails nicely with the concept of bottom-to-top healing (see Figure 7.1).

At its base, Maslow's hierarchy stresses safety and meeting basic physiological needs first before higher order needs may be met. The base of Maslow's pyramid includes core life-sustaining physiological functions. This is similar to the bottom brain functioning of the brain stem, autonomic nervous system, and cerebellum. The middle layers of Maslow's pyramid highlight emotional and safety needs much like the limbic system and midbrain structures in the brain. Finally, the apex of Maslow's hierarchy points to problem solving and factual and creative functions, similar to the prefrontal cortex area of top-brain functions. Like Maslow's model, brain

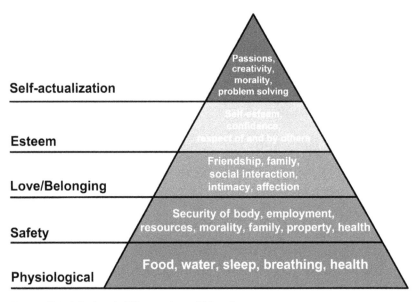

Figure 7.1 Maslow's Hierarchy of Needs

functioning begins at the base with life maintenance functions, and as functional needs are met, it moves upward to executive functions. The trauma-informed counselor must work to help the client establish an initial sense of safety, stability, and predictability, followed by working phases of treatment, including continuing modulation between states of arousal and homeostasis.

Top-level function draws on cortical processes, including language, narrative, and the perception of meaning as applied to life trauma and experiences. Trauma healing bottom to top suggests that brain areas and neural connections beginning with sensory and bodily awareness should optimally connect with top-down functioning including reasoning, planning, memory, and focus skills, and finally culminating in integration.

Case Example

A couple married for seven years came to see a marriage counselor for "poor communication" and extreme dissatisfaction with their marriage. Both initially appeared agitated and engaged in repeated verbal jousting and threw barbs toward each other. Each denied and failed to recognize that their own internal state was triggering fight-or-flight responses during their communication. The counselor's initial treatment objective was to help the couple to reestablish calm and begin to work from bottom to top to quiet their own and their partner's triggered responses and interactions. The counselor introduced and explained how wearing a device called a pulse oximeter (a small noninvasive medical feedback device clasped on the index finger that measures pulse rate and oxygen saturation level of blood) during sessions might help apprise of individual states of physiological hyper-arousal with a fight-or-flight response (Gottman & Gottman, 2010). Their constant state of hyper-arousal during communication was blocking the couple from accessing top cortical brain areas required for problem solving and higher level brain functioning. Yet they both held hope that relationship counseling could help them bring positive change to their relationship. The stoic and avoiding husband was especially surprised when the pulse oximeter pointed to his highly elevated pulse rate, pointing to possible flooding and sympathetic nervous system arousal and stress levels well out of the window of tolerance. The therapist had previously discussed methods of self-soothing and regulation that could be used by either partner when they recognized nervous system hyper-arousal. The therapist allowed time for a break and calm moment in session before further problem-solving discussions, which resulted in a decrease of defensiveness. The counselor encouraged simple touch and eye contact between the couple, as well as quiet moments, as a means toward calm and soothing. This simple touch, hand holding or a soft and steady touch on the knee, can itself help release oxytocin and promote bonding, and perhaps set the stage for creation of new patterns of interaction

Right Brain–Left Brain Integration

Of equal importance for therapist consideration in trauma healing is horizontal, or side-to-side, healing. Here, the distinct functional differences in right brain and left brain are important. In short review of neurological development, consider that in the earliest years of life the right brain hemisphere is more active and developed. The right brain specializes in nonverbal thought, in what's called 'felt sense.' The right brain specializes in facial recognition, along with increased recognition of patterns. Right brain neural connections are mainly responsible for release of the neurohormone oxytocin and subsequent encouragement of social bonding. The right brain hemisphere also gives constant cues and feedback regarding our internal body sensations and status, called interoception. Interoception is considered by some to be a sixth sense. Specifically, in the forebrain area of the anterior insula and anterior cingulate on the right side of the brain is an area primarily involved in emotional and bodily awareness. Recent studies, however, are suggesting that there are differences in each brain hemisphere regarding interoception and awareness of specific emotional states (Craig, 2003).

The left hemisphere appears to be associated more with parasympathetic activity relating to sense of safety, sense of positive affect, approach-type behaviors, and social promoting emotions. The right hemisphere is associated more with sympathetic nervous system activity, including fear, avoidance, or withdrawal; negative affect; and survival emotions such as anxiety.

The therapist can encourage clients toward activities and treatments supporting integration of right hemisphere–left hemisphere functions. Therapies such as Eye Movement Desensitization and Reprocessing, or EMDR, for example, include the use of bilateral stimulation of side-to-side eye movements for treatment of trauma. Somatic, or body-focused, therapies can also help with hemisphere integration functioning. As the right hemisphere has strong involvement with proprioception and interoception and is so strongly involved in felt sense, therapies that encourage new connections between right and left brain can be beneficial to individuals by bringing awareness of body status and by increasing access to the parasympathetic functioning

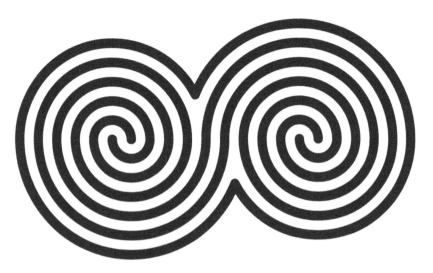

Figure 7.2 Side-by-Side Labyrinth Figure

dominate in left brain. This can be as simple and prescriptive as encouraging a basic walking routine with its crossbody, side-to-side movement. Another tool I have used to encourage bilateral movement and stimulation is called a dual lap labyrinth (see Figure 7.2). This simple device is held on the client's lap and contains a side-by-side labyrinth shape that can be traced with fingers of both hands simultaneously. Clients report this to be soothing, calming, and meditative.

Somatic Connection

Traditionally, preferred methodology for trauma healing has included an emphasis on talk therapy, as the therapist guides clients toward cognitive reasoning to gain clarity and understanding. To put it simply, the trend in therapy has been to access top-down brain functions, including language and talk, in assisting clients to understand and work through experiences of trauma. New findings in neuroscience are pointing to different valuable approaches in the treatment of trauma. New strategies include helping clients connect with right brain–body awareness initially, then pairing it with left brain, more cognitive processes. This helps to bring about increased parasympathetic nervous system function and teaches self-regulation and awareness. Studies are showing that with elevated levels of stress, particularly if chronic and ongoing, complex pathways to cognitive functioning centers may be unavailable. In research cited by the National Academy of Science, "the successful execution of cognitive regulation relies on intact executive functioning and engagement of the prefrontal cortex, both of which are rapidly impaired by the deleterious effects of stress" (Raio et al., 2013, p. 15139). Rather than beginning with cognitive approaches and talk therapy to engage the prefrontal cortex, therapists are looking to the body and body awareness to ease into supporting neural connections; from the motor and afferent nerves throughout the body, spinal cord, and brain stem; through the ever-watchful limbic system; through unique 'spindle' cells of the cingulate cortex; to conscious awareness and memory formations of the hippocampus and the prefrontal cortex. Acknowledging that this is a gross simplification of a complex process, it remains that new neural understanding is suggesting new approaches to healing. This 'somatic first' approach was broadly introduced in 1997 when Peter Levine published his book *Waking the Tiger* (1997). Levine studied physiological responses of animals to environmental threat, noting that animals don't seem to carry stress or stress memory on escaping and surviving the threat. Typically, an animal that survives the attack of a predator will go through a distinct process for recovery, including stabilization of the autonomic nervous system. This may include distinct and involuntary patterns of movement such as shaking followed by deep breathing as the animal reconnects with its body. Levine studied PTSD and chronic stress responses in humans as well, noting that in human autonomic responses to danger, the built-up energy required for escape or response, must also be allowed to be discharged when danger has passed. If such required recovery actions are prevented, the brain continues to signal the release of high levels of cortisol and norepinephrine, leaving body and brain in a chronic state of dysregulation. Symptoms common in PTSD such as nightmares or reenactments are seen as repeated attempts to discharge this frozen energy and return to homeostasis. According to Levine, treatment for trauma should be gentle and gradual, and should "begin to discharge the instinctive survival energy that we did not have a chance to use at the time of an event" (Levine, 2008, p. 31). Levine developed Somatic Experiencing® as a therapeutic treatment approach to conditions like PTSD. For trauma treatment, somatic-focused therapies may provide a gentle and supportive tool allowing the body to discharge energy held since the time of trauma and to return to a state of nervous system regulation and balance. Placing a focus on responses to stress and anxiety is a door through which healing can occur.

Resourcing

In order to facilitate healing, the brain-wise therapist will help the client to identify resources and personal assets to draw upon regularly to shift focus away from the locked-in, repetitive ruminations and typical patterns of engagement with the stress experience. The new field of positive psychology points out the importance of focusing on internal coping strengths and external social supports to leverage resilience and thriving in the midst of ongoing stress (Seligman, 2002). The counselor can help clients identify memories of sensory experiences of comfort and safety, practice creative visualization and imagery of comfort, or identify actual or potential resources currently at their disposal. Several evidence-based trauma therapies include resourcing as a starting point to further trauma work. For example, the eight-phase process of EMDR, as developed by Francine Shapiro in the 1980s, includes Phase 2, or resource installation (Shapiro, 2001). In resource installation the therapist will first ensure that the client can access memories or calming images of safety prior to or in place of recollection of traumatic specific memories. Another potent resource available to therapists includes helping the client to leverage social–emotional brain pathways and feelings of connection with others. As mentioned, such resourcing may allow release of oxytocin in the brain, which can counteract or offset release of cortisol. Resourcing can encourage a sensory focus on importance of touch as a therapeutic means of nervous system regulation. For example, resourcing for couples in therapy can include education on the importance of simple touch, hand holding, and so on, as a brain-wise method to strengthen attachment. Resourcing can leverage beneficial healing aspects of social connection during disaster and trauma (Seppala, 2012). Commonly, people will attempt to reach out to others in times of widespread stress, both to receive instructional cues regarding lifesaving actions to be taken, and to later provide comfort and assist in self-regulation of emotional arousal after imminent threat has passed.

Personal Meaning and Story

In 2005, I worked in disaster mental health response following the destruction from Hurricane Katrina. Tasked with assisting a small southern community in the immediate hurricane aftermath, the mental health response team followed the interventional approach of Psychological First Aid when assisting those impacted by the disaster. Unlike typical therapeutic interventions in individual trauma treatment, the focus of Psychological First Aid is broader, population based, and community focused (Uhernik &

Husson, 2009). Counselor volunteers were encouraged to take moments to actively listen and to become a container for the narratives and stories of survivors. Social connection during storytelling was important, as survivors visibly relaxed and repeatedly expressed gratitude for volunteers from faraway who sat and listened. There were cohesion and common elements to the stories told by many community members. Expressing grief over their many losses took on an almost mythical wistfulness.

Case Example

The Disaster Mental Health volunteer responder sat next to the older lady in the shelter. With a rhythmic southern drawl, the woman asked the volunteer "Where y'all from?" The volunteer gently told the woman that she was from Colorado, then asked the woman how she and her family had fared through the hurricane. The woman got a faraway look in her eyes and said quietly, "All the way from Colorado to our little town, well God bless you . . . I guess you will never get to see our beautiful trees; they are all gone." The woman then lowered her head and talked about sadness and her personal losses. As the volunteer continued talking with people in the shelter, she repeatedly heard a common theme as people mentioned loss, sadness, and their trees that were no more. The trees were a metaphor for their community and for all they had collectively lost. Storytelling became a resource for healing. People spoke individually about loss, but also about the communal experience of their grief. One after another, survivors expressed emotions over disruption, the impermanence of the natural world, and invariably ending with expression of unity and pride, and with the slightest flicker of hope and moving toward recovery.

Helping clients discover personal meaning and telling their unique story can be a critical step toward healing and integration of traumatic experience. Pointing to that which is shared by the community builds strength and a unity of purpose. Brain-wise, this can often be accomplished through means other than language oriented. The nonverbal right brain works well with images and metaphor, as well as the inner experience of felt sense and emotional expression of the traumatic experience. For this reason, holistic integration can occur through talk therapy alternatives including sensory-based therapies such as the visual arts, photography, color therapy or sense of sound through music, chanting, and drumming; expressive kinesthetic therapies such as dance and theater can become an avenue to tell the story. Counselors Vaz & White (2011) focused on post-traumatic growth in the New Orleans community recovering from Hurricane Katrina. They pointed to community cohesion and what they call "culture-bound protective factors." In New Orleans there exists the strong intergenerational practice of dance, community parade and masking traditions that symbolically and ritually represent a sense of life and rebirth. Poetry and haiku (either self-written or reading a selection of meaningful evocative poems written by others) can help in integration. Journaling and letter writing may also help to access emotional right brain content. The act of writing involves motor neuron and movement, proprioception, and body awareness during the manipulation of the writing tool to paper, as well language access and right hemisphere expression of emotions and feelings. For children and adults as well, play therapy such as sand tray work may be helpful for moments when words fail to express the experience, the memory, or a linear story line.

References

Craig, A.D. (2003). Interoception: The sense of the physiological condition of the body. *Current Opinion in Neurobiology*, 13(4), 500–505. doi: 10.1016/SO959-4388(03)00090-4

Gottman, J., & Gottman, J.S. (2010). *Level 1: Bridging the couples chasm.* Seattle, WA: Gottman Institute.

Levine, P.A. (1997). *Waking the tiger: Healing trauma.* Berkeley: North Atlantic Books.

Levine, P.A. (2008). *Healing trauma: A pioneering program for restoring the wisdom of your body.* Boulder, CO: Sounds True.

Raio, C.M., Orederu, T.A., Palazzolo, L., Shurick, A.A., & Phelps, E.A. (2013, September 10). Cognitive emotion regulation fails the stress test. *Proceedings from the National Academy of Sciences of the United States of America*, 110(37), 15139–15144.

Seligman, M.E.P. (2002). *Authentic happiness: Using the new positive psychology to realize your potential for lasting fulfillment.* New York: Free Press.

Seppala, E. (2012, November 6). How the stress of disaster brings people together: New evidence that men are more likely to cooperate in difficult circumstances. *Scientific American.* (retrieved April 15, 2015 from www.scientificamerican.com)

Shapiro, F. (2001). *Eye movement desensitization and reprocessing* (2nd ed.). New York : The Guilford Press.

Uhernik, J.A., & Husson, M.A. (2009). Psychological first aid: An evidence informed approach for acute disaster behavioral health response. Vistas 2009. *American Counseling Association,* (Article 24, pp. 271–280).

Vaz, K., & White, M. (2011). On being an example of hope: Culture specific responses to recovering from a natural disaster. From a presentation at American Counseling Association Annual Conference: New Orleans, LA. March 25, 2011.

8

PACING COUNSELING WITH THE INTENT TO HEAL

With neuroscience as a guide, the counseling process for working with traumatized clients can be planned, tailored, and optimized. The traumatized client's decision to seek assistance through counseling is often long in the making. Typically, many years pass before a client seeks help, with the person suffering long and needlessly. Many factors may prevent clients from seeking help. It is critical for the therapist to work to establish a therapeutic relationship and sense of trust between client and therapist. When people are traumatized, there is often disruption in patterns of attachment.

The therapeutic relationship between counselor and client can hold the key to reestablishing a sense of safety and trust. Neuroscience findings show the importance of social connection and how neurotransmitters such as oxytocin can counteract, or act in opposition to, stress hormones such as cortisol. *Oxytocin is released when human bonding occurs.* Counseling exchange between therapist and client can be likened to a dance of interaction, with the counselor's intuitive sense heightened and client's nervous system gently calming and even synchronizing with the therapist's. In the brain, mirror neurons respond to cues and to the observation of emotional expression in their clients. Neuroscience findings around the activity of mirror neurons can direct counselors to engage ongoing self-awareness during counseling and awareness of mirroring, including body posture and nonverbal awareness and mirroring of speech patterns such as rate, cadence, and rhythm. The counselor who is watchful and aware of his own internal states of emotion, empathy, and understanding can work to better connect with clients and to model a state of calming presence for their clients. The counselor can be a container or holding place for clients as they learn to gently examine and process painful memories, and connect with the felt sense and somatic experience of trauma.

The trauma therapist must foster empowerment for her clients, supporting and encouraging them toward healing. The therapeutic relationship must work toward collaboration between therapist and client, avoiding differentiation of power in the relationship. According to SAMHSA guidelines for a trauma-informed approach for treatment, "Clients are supported in shared decision making, choice, and goal setting to determine the plan of action they need to heal and move forward" (2014b, p. 11).

Establishing Safety

Creating a safe place for clients seeking to heal from trauma requires the counselor to be thoughtful and aware at every stage of the process. Some of the suggestions made here may seem obvious but still deserve mention. For example, the initial point of contact for clients seeking counseling for trauma is often a voice message or answering service. While common in our culture, initial interactions with technology and not with the human connection of voice and handshake can be a subtle reinforcement of clients' sense of isolation in their suffering. Whenever possible, the counselor should speak with their clients by phone with a warm, calm, and friendly tone of voice. Particular attention to phone voice message cadence and tone is important. While ethical requirements dictate that voice messages must indicate urgent directives to seek immediate assistance if in crisis or emergency, this information may also be presented on voice message technology in a calm and caring manner. When an appointment has been set and the client comes to the initial appointment, the neuroscience-aware counselor will have thoughtfully considered the sensory experience of office space, lighting, color, sound, and perhaps even smell (by subtle calming essential oil in an office diffuser or using a spray bottle with essential oil and purified water for cleansing space between sessions).

Allowing clients to choose where to sit and what type of seating is important. Consideration of the client's individual needs helps also, as adolescents may like soft seating so they can kick off their shoes and curl up. One of the most popular and apparently calming seats for many clients in my office is an old wooden rocking chair. While many clients mention that the firm rocker feels better for their back, sometimes the back-and-forth movement seems to help clients quiet their limbic brain and perhaps gently stimulate the cerebellum during session.

For the trauma client, completing a traditional intake form may be difficult and overwhelming. The counselor may need to pace the intake process to not rush the client. One way for the counselor to help is to assist the client in regaining a sense of control. The client is encouraged to set a signal to indicate when he wishes to stop or when he feels flooded. Even before this, much time and care is spent in discovering resources and support for clients, and to educate clients about typical brain responses during and after trauma. Education for the client around physiological brain responses common in trauma can help to normalize their personal experiences of trauma. This reassures clients that while survival related brain functioning served a protective purpose during trauma, some functions now may be 'stuck' in memory loops and stress hormone overload. In disaster response, normalization of responses is an important tenet of psychological first aid. The frequently quoted comment for acute stress response is that of having "a normal reaction to an abnormal situation." Clients often express relief when they are told that what they are experiencing can be explained with a brain-based focus, and that their experiences are a common way for the healthy brain to respond to environmental stressors.

Continued therapeutic focus on establishing safety includes assessing perceptions of safety, and a self-assessment for subjective bodily experience of current nervous system states. Early introduction of concepts such as rating scales or SUDS (Subjective Units of Distress Scale) can help clients regain a sense of control and an understanding of current levels of nervous system functioning. At the same time, the therapist begins to guide clients toward assessing and establishing resources to help them cope, and toward self-regulating their own state within the arousal threshold. For example, in the eight-phase treatment model of EMDR, Phase 2 focuses on providing and strengthening resources for "containment" of high levels of stress or nervous system arousal (Shapiro, 2001). One resource helps clients use brain-based visualization of a container to hold or to place higher levels of distress. Other resources may include holding imagery of a safe or calm place. Having resource tools will help clients regain a sense of control during the pace of counseling and approach later processing of traumatic memories from a calm, limbic-quieted manner.

Finding Calm . . . Body Awareness

A neuroscience approach in trauma counseling must first include the initial objective of stabilization. Consideration of the typical dynamic interplay between limbic system and prefrontal cortex will help therapists guide clients to experience calm, safety, and groundedness. This is where actions of the anterior cingulate come in. In review, the anterior cingulate physically sits above and over the limbic system area and just below the frontal lobe of the cerebral cortex. The anterior cingulate works like a toggle switch between the fear and emotion detection of limbic system, the hippocampal memory center, and the processing, reasoning center of the cortex. According to neuroscientist Andrew Newburg, the anterior cingulate allows for regulation between emotions such as fear and higher reasoning (Newburg, 2009).

A starting place in trauma therapy for calming excessive arousal states and allowing for integration of brain functions is present moment body focus. The therapist can help clients simply notice the sensation of connection—the places where they physically feel contact with the ground. The therapist may suggest, for example, that clients notice the area on the bottom of the feet where their feet touch the floor. If clients are sitting, the therapist can have them notice where different parts of their body touch the chair, such as their back, the backs of the thighs, or the buttocks. The therapist can suggest that the client stand or stretch arms out wide while simultaneously noticing the connection with the floor. Alternatively, the therapist may introduce the concept of body scan, where the attention is directed to various areas of the body to simply make note of sensation or feeling in these areas. A basic progressive relaxation exercise, in which the client is directed to first tighten and then relax various muscle groups, can help the client increase awareness of the body, quiet the mind, and reconnect with sense of safety and stability. The therapist can also guide the client to focus on a specific area of the body (however small or isolated) that feels relaxed, or neutral, or that has an absence of pain. The therapist can suggest that the client rub her hands together briskly (activating flow of energy) and then place the hands upon this area of the body and massage gently, or simply notice the feeling of heat from the hands to this area.

As an adjunct to somatic awareness work in therapy, the counselor may suggest the client attend a yoga or tai chi class. The slow movement, body focus of such a class works to bring back a sense of connectedness, quieting the mind and grounding the body. Some clients may find a weight training class can help to focus awareness on the body and to improve overall cognitive functioning (Ramirez & Kravitz, 2012). Yoga and tai chi will be discussed in detail in Chapter 9.

Moving to Top Brain: Cognitive Treatment Approaches

The overriding goal of therapeutic interventions in trauma treatment has been the restoration of nervous system regulation and homeostasis, which allows higher level reasoning and future problem solving to occur, unhindered by emotions and flooding. Therapists and counselors, as modern-day healers, have depended on, in varying degrees, the ability of the traumatized person to articulate through language, their emotions, memories, and perceptions. So-called talk therapy has been the treatment modality of choice in the past. Talk therapy is dependent on adequate functioning and neural connections of the language and processing areas of the brain. Broca's area and Wernicke's and surrounding areas are located in most people in the left frontal cortex area of the brain (although in a small percentage of left-handed people, these language areas are found in the right hemisphere; Carter et al., 2014). As we have seen, neural connections from lower brain stem and limbic areas can take control or temporarily 'hijack' functions from higher brain areas in moments of perceived danger, and moments that require immediate survival actions. The memory center interacts through recall of similar past experiences of danger and protects based on past memory by thwarting an ill-advised response. This leaves language and processing centers of the brain playing catch-up. When treatment 'success' depends first on ability to express and process in words and higher level reasoning, the possibility of integration and improved functioning is decreased. As mentioned previously, the therapist of today is increasingly helping clients quiet autonomic nervous system responses and calm the ever-vigilant limbic system. Sometimes this treatment alone can be of great assistance to clients with PTSD, or with those who remain in a continuing state of hyper-arousal, or even those with hypo-arousal with protective dissociation or shutdown.

However, if the therapist can help guide clients toward self-regulation and more balanced nervous system functioning, attention can then focus on top-brain functions and integration.

Cognitive behavioral therapies, with focus on recognizing and changing thought patterns, can be helpful later in the therapeutic process. Other trauma treatments that highlight movement toward top-brain functioning include the variations on cognitive behavioral therapy(s). Cognitive behavioral therapy recognizes that thoughts help mediate and interpret between changing environmental or situational demands. Thoughts also influence attempts to respond to demands, and changing behavioral response patterns may in turn influence beliefs about self. Acceptance of altered beliefs about self and incorporating new patterns of learning are desired outcomes in cognitive behavioral therapy (SAMSHA, 2014a). There are many variations of cognitive behavioral interventions that have been researched and are effectively used in the later phases of treatment of trauma.

Some therapeutic interventions, however, have been questioned regarding efficacy, particularly when used as an immediate intervention or in acute stress disorder stage.

The popular intervention of Critical Incident Stress Debriefing (CISD), for example, relies on early and immediate intervention following a trauma incident. This includes the intent to provide 'closure' for persons impacted by the trauma. It is a facilitator-led intervention directed toward groups immediately impacted by a traumatic event. Participants are encouraged to 'talk' about their experiences and memories within the group, with a highlight on verbalizing the sensory aspects recalled after the trauma incident. There are now controlled studies indicating that this early top-brain-focused intervention, while well-intentioned, might actually impede subsequent natural neural progression toward healing (McNally et al., 2003). For example, certain components of CISD, such as allowing or encouraging groups of people the opportunity to be together for comfort and support of each other, may activate an autonomic quieting and bonding. Mirror neurons can be activated when social groups are allowed to connect and demonstrate caring and support for each person in the group. Avoiding verbal reexperiencing of the event would be important, however, to help avoid contagion of emotional, limbic responses and shutting down of cognitive processes. Perhaps neuroscience can point to new understanding of how to assist people in regaining equilibrium, and move through phases of acute stress following trauma toward resiliency and health. Future research in neuroscience may help point to a different staging of interventions and leveraging best healing options.

Other top-brain approaches that can effectively be used after teaching clients to regulate lower brain functions include cognitive processing models such as 'exposure therapies' and other modalities such as Cognitive Processing Therapy (CPT). CPT asks clients to write a detailed account of the trauma experience that includes thoughts, sensory perceptions, and emotions. Clients are then encouraged to read aloud their written narrative of the event during session. Clients are then directed to identify faulty beliefs and cognitive distortions in interpretation of the event (Resick & Schnicke, 1992). Exposure therapy directs the client to repeatedly describe and consider memories, specific objects, and places of the trauma, and to experience the intense emotions that may accompany such recollection. Then the recollections are repeatedly brought to mind in a carefully monitored manner until there is an eventual decrease in arousal and sympathetic nervous system activation with memories of the event. The use of exposure therapy has been shown to be an effective trauma treatment with certain clients (Rothbaum et al., 2000) but has potential to cause a worsening of symptoms and adverse effects in other clients. It also should only be used by the therapist having adequate training.

Other cognitive or top-brain therapies include narrative therapies, which can guide clients to examine their own unique and also societal parameters of their trauma experience. Existential philosophical approaches focus on helping the client understand the meaning of suffering and implications and changes that suffering has brought into life. Other treatment approaches, such as the well-researched evidence-based EMDR, use some component of helping correct cognitive distortions of trauma. EMDR will be examined in Chapter 9 as an integrative therapy for trauma.

References

Carter, R., Aldridge, S., Page, M., & Parker, S. (2014). *The human brain book* (2nd ed.). New York: DK Publishing.

McNally, R.J., Bryant, R.A., & Ehlers, A. (2003). Does early psychological intervention promote recovery from posttraumatic stress? *Psychological Science in the Public Interest, 4*, 45–79.

Newburg, A.B. (2009). *How God changes your brain: Breakthrough findings from a leading neuroscientist.* New York: Ballantine Books.

Ramirez, A., & Kravitz, L. (2012). Resistance training improves mental health. *IDEA Fitness Journal*, 9(1), 20–22. (retrieved April 16, 2015 from www.unm.edu/~lkravitz/Article%20 folder/RTandMentalHealth.html)

Resick, P.A., & Schnicke, M.K. (1992). Cognitive processing therapy for sexual assault victims. *Journal of Consulting and Clinical Psychology*, 60, 748–756.

Rothbaum, B.O., Meadows, E.A., Resick, P., & Foy, D.W. (2000). Cognitive-behavioral therapy. In Foa, E.B., & Keane, T.M. (Eds.), *Effective treatments for PTSD: Practice guidelines from the International Society for Traumatic Stress Studies* (pp. 60–83). New York: Guilford Press.

Shapiro, F. (2001). *Eye movement desensitization and reprocessing: Basic principles, protocols, and procedures* (2nd ed.). New York: Guilford Press.

Substance Abuse and Mental Health Services Administration. (2014a). *SAMHSA's concept of trauma and guidance for a trauma-informed approach. HHS Publication No.* 14-4884 (SMA). Rockville, MD: Substance Abuse and Mental Health Services Administration.

Substance Abuse and Mental Health Services Administration. (2014b). *Trauma-informed care in behavioral health services: (TIP) Series 57. HHS Publication No.* (SMA) 14–4816. Rockville, MD: Substance Abuse and Mental Health Services Administration.

THE WHOLE OF EXPERIENCE

Integrative and Creative Approaches for Trauma Treatment

Neuroscience discoveries, in tandem with a renewed interest in healing practices of other cultures, considers body-based approaches of Eastern cultures as one method of healing and a return to balanced states of neurological functioning. As we have discovered, our brains and bodies function together in a continuous dance of interaction. Our bodies carry out the movement and directives of the brain, but also have reflexive actions, thought-free motions that protect us from harm. For example, with properly functioning afferent and motor neurons in the fingertips, we automatically draw back after touching a hot stove, even before the brain has time to remember that we might have left the burner on. Embedded within the language of our culture are numerous references to mind–body connections. Consider the following common expressions: "I didn't have the heart to tell him," "I felt it in my gut, but I just didn't listen," "He/she is a pain in the neck," "I choked up," and "My heart was in my throat." These and many more are language-based expressions acknowledging the interaction of emotions, mind, and body. The alert therapist can assist clients in exploring these linguistic expressions further, perhaps with a nudge toward increasing awareness of trauma blocks and of somatic memories of trauma experiences.

This chapter will highlight integrative approaches, with confirmation from neuroscience findings that can be used for treatment of trauma. These approaches can be used as stand-alone and/or referral sources, or, with proper training of the counselor, as adjunct to traditional counseling approaches.

Somatic Approaches

Yoga, based on an ancient philosophy, is described as "an in-depth training in participatory observation and enhancement of the body, heart and mind" (Powers, 2008, p. 3). While there are many different types of yoga, some emphasizing the physical postures or poses of yoga, others emphasizing the movement through the poses, still others are considered restorative or gentle yoga (Hanley, 2015). All types of yoga focus on the breath (known as prana or 'life force'). When attention is drawn to the breath, autonomic nervous system functions lean to parasympathetic balance, the mind quiets and calms. A practice of yoga can be of immense benefit for clients who have trauma. In a randomized controlled study, a short-term yoga practice among a group of women experiencing chronic, previously untreatable PTSD resulted in a significant reduction in trauma symptoms (van der Kolk, 2015).

While yoga can be highly recommended as an adjunct for ongoing trauma therapy and treatment, the yoga-trained therapist can also introduce specific yoga postures during therapy session that can provide specific energetic balancing for symptoms as they arise.

Case Example

Andrea is a 36-year-old woman coming to counseling to learn tools to help her better manage anxiety and enjoy her relationship with her husband.

In a previous marriage Andrea had experienced domestic violence. With help and counseling support,

Andrea had been able to leave the marriage and establish a new life. She learned to recognize when she felt triggered and anxious. She had learned in therapy tools to help with affect regulation and soothing. She also learned about safety and to recognize patterns of relationship violence. She wanted to strengthen her new-found sense of self-worth and empowerment.

During session, she spoke of the feeling in her body when her thoughts turn to memories of "I am weak and I am defenseless." To help reestablish her sense of safety and stability, the office coffee table was moved aside and the client began to focus on breathing and on a standing yoga pose of strength, connection, and groundedness. Initial moments were spent in yoga Mountain Pose and then gentle movements toward the strong and steady Warrior Pose (Figure 9.1) were achieved.

Andrea experienced a moment of empowerment, strong and firm presence and awareness of her body,

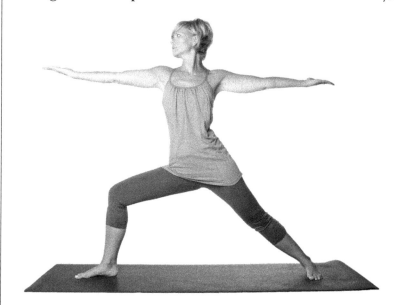

Figure 9.1 Yoga Warrior Pose

and an increase in clarity of mind. She also learned a
tool that she could take away from session and use when
needed for support, as well as gaining a strong desire to
begin her own regular yoga practice.

While yoga is a practice that can be encouraged by the
trauma therapist as an adjunct to ongoing trauma therapy
work, other body-based trauma therapy modalities are
beginning to receive research focus. One of these is based
on the work of Peter Levine called Somatic Experiencing,
or SE®. SE® is a trauma treatment modality that guides the
client to focus on internal physiological states including proprioception (awareness of musculo-skeletal functioning)
and interoception (awareness of internal organ functioning
such as heartbeat and lung functions). The primary goal of
SE® is to help to relieve the debilitating symptoms of trauma
and chronic stress. Somatic experiencing looks at trauma
from a neurological perspective by focusing on bottom-up
interventions to help quiet states of dysregulation. According to Levine, somatic experiencing works by "approaching
the charged memories indirectly and very gradually" and by
"facilitating the generation of new corrective interoceptive
experiences that contradict those of overwhelm and help-
lessness" (Payne et al., 2015, p. 1). Somatic experiencing
does not require that a person revisit memories of trauma
for processing, nor does it require verbal processing around
traumatic experience. Rather, it focuses on physiological
experience in the current moment. While research has not
yet focused specifically on somatic treatment modalities
per se, ongoing research is focused on the concept of interoception. Interoception appears linked in the brain from
the insular and anterior cingulate cortices to the prefrontal cortex. Through the neural connections in these areas
comes a sense of self and an awareness of internal bodily

functioning. Other somatic-based trauma therapies have helped to provide a conceptual model for understanding of autonomic regulation processes. The work of Pat Ogden (Ogden et al., 2006) expands on the concept of 'window of tolerance' first described by Dan Siegel (1999). In Ogden's sensorimotor psychotherapy, maintaining a balanced and regulated state of autonomic nervous system functioning within a range between hyper-arousal and hypo-arousal is the goal. When ANS functioning is within the window of tolerance, the client can begin to process and find resolution to traumatic memories and experience.

An ancient approach to mind–body healing can be found in the practice of tai chi and qi gong. The practice of qi gong dates back over 5,000 years in Chinese history. Tai chi, which holds many similarities to qi gong, developed more recently. In both, the practitioner engages in a series of slow purposeful movements. The Chinese refer to these as having a threefold focus known as the 'three regulations.' Included are a body focus (including smooth, flowing movements and emphasis on posture), a focus on the breath, and a mind focus (showing familiarity to mindful awareness similar to Western techniques of mindfulness). Both tai chi and qi gong have been shown through randomized controlled trials to foster a quieting of neurohormonal sympathetic nervous system response (Jahnke et al., 2010). Specifically, tai chi practice has been shown to improve heart rate and decrease blood levels of neurohormones epinephrine and norepinephrine. Qi gong practice has been shown to decrease these blood levels of epinephrine and also of circulating cortisol levels. Both modalities can be offered to trauma clients to help them to return to a more balanced state of autonomic nervous system functioning, either prior to or concurrent to trauma therapy treatment.

In the 1970s, Harvard Medical School physician Herbert Benson developed a treatment model he termed the 'relaxation response.' Drawing upon studies of the meditation practice known as transcendental meditation, Benson included a progressive focus on relaxation of various parts of the body combined with focus and attention drawn to the breath (Benson, 2015). Benson originally wrote his best-selling book *The Relaxation Response* in 1975 and has continued to study the benefits of meditation for physiological and mental well-being.

As mentioned in previous chapters, a basic and fundamental technique for helping clients self-regulate autonomic nervous system functioning is to teach methods that focus on the breath (Novotny & Kravitz, 2007).

Diaphragmatic breathing, unilateral forced nostril breathing, and methods of breathing taught in the practice of yoga are great starting points for clients. Another breathing method especially suited to tapping into autonomic nervous system functions is referred to as ratio breathing. Physiologically, the act of breathing includes the ongoing state of balance between slight sympathetic nervous system activation on the inhalation phase and the slowing, calming exhalation phase activation of the parasympathetic nervous system. A slight deliberate lengthening of the exhalation phase of the breath can help shift the autonomic nervous system out of a state of sympathetic dominance and support parasympathetic functioning. Teaching clients awareness and breath focus has the dual advantage of physiologically promoting calm and developing an intrinsic sense of empowerment and belief in the ability to self-heal.

Energy Psychology

There are therapies for treatment of trauma that fall into the emerging area of what is known as energy psychology (EP). Even though these therapies are based on healing methods of ancient origin, Western medicine has been hesitant to embrace these integrative therapies or often dismisses them due to lack of controlled research trials and apparent inability to explain the mechanism of action. Commonly, energy psychology focuses on a relationship of energy systems and interactions between mind and body, including the electrical activity of brain and nervous system, the heart, and areas of the body known in Eastern medicine as meridians. Research, including neurobiology, is pointing to the usefulness of EP as a helpful adjunct to conventional trauma treatment. For example, a study was done in an orphanage in Rwanda with 50 young survivors of genocide. The EP modality of Thought Field Therapy was used in a single 20- to 30-minute session with resulting dramatic relief from long standing symptomatology of PTSD in survivors. These results proved long lasting, demonstrated by follow-up assessments after a year (Sakai et al., 2010). In addition, there is a current research project at Harvard Medical School that is using neuroimaging to detect limbic system changes following use of acupuncture as a treatment modality. There are over 30 variations of EP techniques in use that go by various names, including Thought Field Therapy, Emotional Freedom Technique, or Tapping. Many techniques do have several things in common. Most include (1) the client bringing to mind a thought or memory stressor (which can include either distressing material or a potentially positive stressor like performance anxiety) and (2) the client holding this stressor as a short imaginal exposure while simultaneously tapping on certain acupoints similar to the acupuncture points in Chinese medicine. In studies cited by David Feinstein (2010), there is increasing support for use of energy psychology in treatment of trauma. There is often a significant reduction in autonomic nervous system arousal reported after a short session, making it a helpful addition for Cognitive Behavioral Therapy and other standard trauma treatment modalities. Other EP modalities focus on the nonphysical energy fields surrounding the body and present in all living things—as described by many cultures—and are similar to concept of 'chi' in ancient Chinese culture, 'prana' in Indian culture, and 'life force' for many indigenous people. Reiki, a healing modality that holds the concept of 'ki,' involves a nonmanipulative, gentle energy focus moving through the healer to the client and works to clear energy blockages within body systems. Somewhat similar to Reiki are the energy healing methods known as Therapeutic Touch or Healing Touch. These techniques are often advocated by the profession of nursing and show promise for pain management, soothing and calming. While therapists are usually not trained in these modalities, and may or may not be likely to include these in their practice, they can nevertheless learn about these techniques and provide support for their clients. There is also support for encouraging therapists and other care providers to pay attention to their own stress and to learn trauma release through methods of self-care. Hospital teams, for example, are increasingly making EP modalities available at the worksite to provide comfort for the stress-burdened caregivers (NPR, 2015).

Case Example

Stacy, a 32-year-old woman, came to see an energy psychology focused therapist because she was struggling to cope with chronic generalized anxiety and panic disorder stretching back to her childhood. She noticed a recent elevation of levels of anxiety, which now included occasional, nonspecific suicidal ideation. Stacy denied that she was actively suicidal, pointing to her desire to complete nursing school and begin her career in nursing. The therapist initially explained the concept of a rating scale (0–10) for levels of anxiety, including information that higher anxiety scale levels typically correspond to lower levels of functioning of the prefrontal cortex. Stacy was taught how to self-soothe and use methods to bring down her anxiety rating score. Tools to calm current anxiety levels included feet mindfulness, a meditative method for mind focus and energy shift. Feet mindfulness taught the client to draw her attention to the bodily area of the feet such that the energy pooled in her head was drawn down through her lungs and abdomen, all the way to her feet. She allowed herself to imagine breathing in and out the palms of her feet, and then to notice her decrease in ruminating thoughts, all while staying focused and grounded through her feet. The therapist also used Tapping on energy meridians as tool to further decrease her elevated anxiety levels.

The therapist next turned to helping Stacy address social anxiety. From an energy psychology approach, the therapist determined that this client was 'energy sensitive,' an empath and intuitive. This therapist used a drawing of a consciousness map to clarify and assist Stacy in better understanding the people around her and in better understanding her intuitive assessment of the values and motivations of those around her. Energetic boundaries were explored, including how to feel and sense her boundaries and how to set firm boundaries with others. Through therapy, Stacy was able to better manage her anxiety and complete her oral presentation for a final nursing exam.

Another area of research on mind–body interaction with implications for trauma treatment focuses on heart rate variability (HRV). Medical science, particularly the field of cardiology, has long noted the connection between the nervous system and the heart. Vagal nerve functions of the autonomic nervous system have direct and ongoing impact on the heart. Psychological and emotional states can affect the autonomic nervous system and, in turn, the regulation and function of the heart. Heart rate variability basically describes the length of time between heartbeats. It is physiologically important for the heart to have the ability to adapt to the constantly changing requirements of the environment and internal states. There is continuous interplay between sympathetic nervous system responses and parasympathetic nervous system influences on the actions of the heart (Friedman & Thayer, 1998). For optimal health, the heart needs to have higher levels of heart rate variability. Assisting clients in learning to self-regulate their autonomic nervous system can help clients return to healthier states of functioning. Heart rate variability can be detected and relayed back to the client through various biofeedback monitoring devices. The client can use simple breathing techniques that may bring about a quieting of sympathetic influences along with HRV feedback confirmation of the progress being made. There are a number of such HRV feedback devices available including apps for smart phones and computers. The therapist will benefit from learning about HRV and passing along information and understanding to clients in support of efforts to learn mind–body approaches.

Another EP-related tool for treatment of trauma includes the field of aromatherapy. The direct link between nerve endings in each nostril direct to the olfactory bulb on the corresponding side deep within the limbic system makes our sense of smell the most immediate and evocative of our senses. Certain scents may evoke memories and emotional associations for clients. The field of aromatherapy posits that certain essences or elements of certain plants may be distilled or processed to extract what are called essential oils. The use of plant essences in treatment of physical and emotional conditions goes back to prehistoric times. Earliest written histories point to use of parts of plants such as roots, leaves, flowers, bark, and fruits being used for medicinal purposes. Many of the pharmaceutical medications in use today were derived from various plants. These include bark from a species of willow tree that produces salicin. Salicin was used as a pain reliever and anti-blood-clotting agent and was later processed to be used as what is commonly known as aspirin. Historically, all drugs were derived from natural substances. Many world cultures draw from a plant basis of medicine. The Ayurvedic system of medicine still used today in India is believed to be over 5,000 years old. Use of herbs and plant medicines is a part of ancient Chinese culture as well, with a written drug directory dating from 2,800 years ago. The utility of such systems of medicine is beginning to be blended into current Western medicine traditions.

Essential oils are obtained by a process that extracts from parts of certain plants the healing essence of these plants. This process usually includes distillation or extreme pressure applied to the plant parts to squeeze out the oil. The chemical components of essential oils can be analyzed by modern tools of mass spectography. It is estimated that there are more than half a million species of plants in the world, and of these only about 300 are used for modern practice of aromatherapy (Worwood, 1996). Various plant parts may be used to extract essential oils. Most people have had the pleasant emotional and sensual experience of direct inhalation of a rose flower, for example.

The use of essential oils and the general field of aromatherapy is being given a new look as an adjunct and special tool for treatment of emotional and behavioral health conditions such as depression and anxiety disorders. It is important that a counselor obtain training in proper use of essential oils in a counseling setting. Aromatherapy may be used as an adjunct to therapy at all phases of a general treatment plan. Beginning with the therapist as she prepares for seeing scheduled clients, the therapist may select an essential oil to briefly inhale in a moment of mindful awareness and centering of her own nervous system prior to interaction with their clients. Depending on intake knowledge of presenting concerns of specific clients, an essential oil may be diffused and sprayed in office space of the therapist. While individual responses and preferences toward specific essential oils may vary and always should be systematically assessed, surrounding the office environment with a calming fragrance to start the day of seeing clients can help to soothe and ground both client and therapist. Scents that are universally accepted to be calming and soothing, such as rose and lavender, can be used in combination with distilled water and spritzed as a room freshener. At the beginning of case conceptualization, individual clients can be given the opportunity to sample and discover essential oil essences that they are especially drawn to, and these oils may be provided in small amounts carried for inhalation and used to soothe and provide nervous system self-regulation. Knowledge of diagnostic nuances of the client may be helpful in determining specific essential oils for each client. There are specific essential oils that are commonly used for elevated anxiety levels and hyper-arousal of the nervous system. These may include lavender, neroli, rose otto, frankincense, patchouli, and more. Specific oils, such as lavender or frankincense, may be helpful during episodes of panic attacks. Low energy states and hypo-arousal of the nervous system may be helped with citrus-related oils such as bergamot, lemon, neroli, and geranium. For trauma clients who during therapy may experience dissociated states, oil of peppermint may be used for inhalation to assist clients to stay present and grounded during treatment. While use of essential oils is generally considered safe and is noninvasive, education for clients on best use is imperative. The therapist should seek aromatherapy training, preferably from a certified aromatherapist. Use of essential oils in therapy and instruction to clients for continuing use post treatment may provide a bridge and tool to connect from therapy room to day-to-day experience.

Neurobiological Modalities

Neurobiological modalities for mental health and trauma treatment include EMDR, Brainspotting, neurofeedback, and more. In the treatment of trauma, or mental health in general, few techniques have received more attention and research than EMDR. Developed by Francine Shapiro in the late 1980s, EMDR has received attention and recommendation for the treatment of PTSD. The American Psychological Association has deemed EMDR a grade level A treatment for PTSD (DeAngelis, 2008). According to EMDR founder Francine Shapiro, "Studies show that the eye movements utilized in EMDR are correlated with a desensitizing effect, an increase in parasympathetic activity, and a decrease in psychophysiological arousal" (Solomon & Shapiro, 2008, p. 322). EMDR is an eight-phase protocol that includes early history taking and installing of positive resource imagery prior to the reprocessing phases. The early phases of EMDR are highly applicable to any client, whether the treatment planning is trauma informed or not. Providing clients with specific resources including visualization and mindful awareness can be valuable for all. Resource installation alone can be used for general stress reduction and proactive management and regulation of emotions. EMDR uses bilateral stimulation (side-to-side eye movements, bilateral auditory tones, or tactile pulses), simultaneously with short intervals during which the client brings distressing memories to mind. The client is asked to verbalize any negative belief she may hold about self in regard to the traumatic memory. A rating scale called a SUDS score (subjective units of distress scale) is given with a range of 0 to 10 (with 10 the highest distress level). The client will also identify a positive or desired belief or cognition. A further rating scale is used to rate the strength of belief or validity of the client's positive cognition. Research continues to explore the working mechanism behind EMDR. Some researchers believe that the lateral eye movements may somehow disrupt intensity and accompanying emotional distress experienced during brief exposure of the traumatic memory. Others point to the similarities between bilateral eye movements during the processing stage and the sleep stage of rapid eye movement. There are specific training requirements and supervision hours necessary for the therapist who wishes to obtain EMDR certification.

A newer brain-based therapy known as Brainspotting originally evolved as an extension from EMDR. According to psychologist David Grand, founder of Brainspotting, this tool for working with trauma uses "the strengths of brain-based and talk therapy into a powerful technique to help to heal" (Grand, 2013, p. 169). Grand highlights the importance of the therapeutic relationship between therapist and client, encouraging the therapist to "attune" to both the client and the client's brain processes. The latter is accomplished by close observation of the direction of the client's gaze and reflexive responses during verbal recounting of traumatic memories. The basic theory behind Brainspotting is that where we look or orient can provide information about what is going on in our brains. This new methodology is just beginning to gain research attention and focus. At this point, however, clinicians can be aware of this possible tool and watchful for research findings on efficacy for Brainspotting as a neurobiological approach to trauma healing.

Expressive Therapies

Throughout this book we have mentioned how traditional talk therapy may fall short in the treatment of trauma. Clients are often best served by therapists who are able to bring an eclectic or multimodal approach to their work or, at the least, who can ethically provide adjunct referrals to professionals in other areas. Having experience or training in expressive therapies may give a substantial boost to therapeutic progress made by clients and provide clients with tools for continuing growth and healing throughout their life. There are many different forms of expressive therapies with an estimated 30,000 trained practitioners specializing in the field (Malchiodi, 2005). A common factor with the many expressive therapies is action. Expressive therapies usually include some action on the part of clients. In addition, expressive therapies are sensate and draw on individual experience of the world, inner experience, and memory re-creation.

Of all expressive therapies, music therapy has seemed to have the greatest link to neuroscience research. This appears to be true, judging from quantifiable responses in the brain exposed to music, whether through participatory activities or by the measuring of physiological processes. According to the American Association of Music Therapy (n.d.), music therapy exists as "an established profession in which music is used within a therapeutic relationship to address physical, emotional, cognitive and social needs of individuals." Brain-wise, the regularity and rhythmicity of sound is initially detected through the auditory cortex, and exposure stimulates both the cerebellum and connections back and forth to the frontal cortex. Music research has also pointed to the connecting brain region of the limbic system and to the brain center area of the ventral striatum, specifically that of the nucleus accumbens. The nucleus accumbens is believed to be part of the brain's reward system, which plays a role in experience of pleasure, as well as in addiction (Levitin, 2006). There are innovative ways in which the trauma therapist can point his client to music as a therapeutic adjunct for treatment of trauma. In 2008, a research study provided music workshop training to mental health professionals followed by group music therapy for young male soldiers suffering from PTSD (Bensimon et al., 2008). In this study, soldiers participated in group drumming sessions. Study results showed increased levels of social connection and sense of belonging; increased association with traumatic memories within a safe environment for expression, allowing expression of rage through loudness or cadence of sound of drums; and increased self-efficacy and mastery of rhythms both simple and complex.

In my counseling office I have a medium-sized single drum. At times the drum is adopted by clients, particularly adolescent male clients, and used as a tool for bilateral stimulation and calming or simply as an activity during which simultaneous talking and drumming may ensue. Drumming can be encouraged in group settings as a means to strengthen social cohesion and a sense of belonging, and to draw on attachment. Other methods of incorporating music can include song or chant. Particularly with children, simple, familiar melodies can be re-created with their own words of comfort or reassurance. Clients may be asked to bring to session a favorite piece of music that is calming for them, which they can share and play at the beginning of session. Music therapy research can provide a guide to music suggestions based on rhythm or beats per minute, which has been shown to match with a slowing of heart rate and activation of the parasympathetic nervous system. Specifically, researchers found that exposure to certain pieces of music could reduce heart rate and increase the depth of respiration (Bernardi et al., 2009). Interestingly, researchers noted that these physiological responses to music exposure were similar among participants, whether they reportedly liked the piece of music or not.

There are myriad ways in which art can be incorporated into trauma therapy work. Referrals can be made to therapists who have certification in the field of art therapy. According to Collie et al. (2006, p. 158), "Non-verbal expression as is used in art therapy can facilitate both the shift to declarative memory and the creation of a coherent narrative." Art therapy has been used with many different trauma clients, including victims of sexual abuse and domestic violence, combat veterans, and victims of war and terrorism. Neuroscience suggests that art modalities used for treatment of trauma are helpful by allowing expression of traumatic memories in a nonlinguistic manner and by using expressive art as a container for frightening material. Using art modalities for treatment may increase self-esteem or pride in accomplishment and increase relaxation during process with accompanying reduction in nervous system arousal.

Art therapy may also involve bilateral hemispheres of the brain, particularly when nondominant and dominant hands are both used. Therapists can find more information about certification and board credentialed art therapists though the Art Therapy Credential Board (www.atcb.org) or the American Art Therapy Association.

A recent and compelling project involving art as therapy involved having veterans create masks (National Geographic, 2015). These soldiers created painted masks that symbolically represented themes such as death, pain, and patriotism. The symbolic and insightful creations of this project spoke of each participating veteran's strong and powerful movement toward personal healing from trauma.

There is also recent popular culture interest in the use of coloring and drawing, particularly aimed toward adults seeking soothing methods for stress relief and relaxation. There are coloring books available with geometric shapes and nature-related scenes that can be adapted and made available during therapy sessions for clients to color, even during conversation with the therapist or as directed during imaginal moments. In her book *Tapping In,* EMDR therapist Laura Parnell (2008) suggests using drawing imagery of a peaceful or safe place along with bilateral stimulation as a tool to help clients learn self-regulation of the autonomic nervous system. Years ago, Carl Jung suggested the use of a particular type of drawing known as a mandala to be used therapeutically with clients. Mandalas are circular or square shapes that always point to the center area wherein may be found an interpretation or representation of the Self. Jung reportedly suggested mandala drawing for his patients, but also for himself noting, "I sketched every morning in a notebook a small circular drawing, a mandala, which seemed to correspond to my inner situation at the time. With the help of these drawings I could observe my psychic transformations from day to day" (Jung, 1965, p. 195). A recent study by researchers at Texas A&M and Emory University School of Medicine looked at using mandala drawing as a tool for stress reduction in individuals suffering from PTSD (Henderson et al., 2007). A group of 36 PTSD subjects were divided into two groups and were instructed to draw either a personal mandala (not using a preset patterned mandala outline) or an unspecified object. Participants were instructed to draw for 20-minute intervals for three days in a row. Those in the mandala group showed a measureable decrease in PTSD symptoms at one month follow-up as compared to those who drew an object. Perhaps a salient factor included the opportunity to express personal symbols and emotional associations with trauma into the personal mandalas. Other studies are suggesting that mandala drawing may be useful with mild levels of stress as well.

Journaling, or expressive writing, is a commonly prescribed therapeutic tool and integrative therapy modality. Many variations of expressive writing techniques are encouraged; however, there is a shortage of research pointing to efficacy of using writing as a trauma treatment tool. Some studies show that using short-term expressive writing can have a positive effect on immune system functioning (Pennebaker & Seagal, 1999). However, some subjects also reported a worsening of mood in the immediate hours after writing. Expressive writing may be therapeutic when combined in later stages of trauma treatment with creation of personal narrative and meaning. As brain functions following trauma treatment tip toward top-down and side-to-side functioning, the powerful addition of words and language expressed through writing may lead to healing and resolution. Recommendations for reading or writing poetry may also foster healing, as clients sort through and find meaning in personal struggle. Use of metaphor, as is often found in poetic expression, may be a particularly powerful method of healing, understanding, and integration. Chapter 7 discussed the importance of the expression of personal narrative and meaning as an integral part of recovery and healing of trauma. Telling the story, whether through writing, storytelling, or other expressive arts, can be an effective method to move past trauma and toward healing.

Mindfulness, Visualization, Affirmation

The concept of mindfulness has become a prominent motif in psychotherapy and trauma treatment. Two basic tenets of mindfulness include being present in the moment and accepting without judgment the thoughts, emotions, and observations that may arise. Learning to be mindful and aware of the present moment often involves a major shift for many people, particularly in our culture. Our fast-paced, future-oriented, outward-focused society tends not to place value on inward reflection, or on gentle acceptance of personal experience, particularly that which is perceived as unpleasant. Inclusion of mindfulness-based interventions in the treatment of trauma appears to have value (Follette et al., 2006). Mindfulness during trauma therapy may help the client maintain a dual focus of awareness. As described by Siegel (2010), dual focus of awareness helps clients to maintain "one focus of awareness on the here and now, another on the there and then" (p. 162). A mindful sense of presence in the moment helps clients to quiet states of hyper-arousal, and may decrease dissociative responses upon reexposure to trauma memory fragments. It also may encourage clients to break from habitual patterns of avoidance and engage more fully in therapy.

Visualization is defined as a "technique involving focusing on positive mental images in order to achieve a particular goal" ("Visualization," n.d.). Visualization or imagery techniques are part of many trauma treatment modalities. In EMDR, visualization on positive images of safety, calm, and nurturing can become a resource for clients during the difficult work of memory reprocessing. These positive resources can be consciously brought to awareness as part of a dual focus approach. Positive imagery may include visualization of a place of calm and comfort, of a nurturing figure available to soothe, or a of mythic figure of strength and protection. Visualization techniques may also evoke an image of a container to use to safely lock away disturbing thoughts or material. Visualization is often used with future focus on success and desired goals or accomplishment. Visualization can be taught and used by any clients wishing to increase resilience, manage stress, or enhance well-being.

Use of positive affirmations as a creative tool and therapy adjunct is also a part of many trauma therapy protocols. In the energy psychology method of Tapping, or Emotional Freedom Technique, dual awareness is held with the distressing thoughts expressed simultaneously with a positive statement of affirmation (Feinstein, 2012). Variations usually include the development of the affirmation statement to include the following: "Even though _____ [fill in the blank with summary words of the distressing situation, thought, or memory] . . . I completely accept myself." The affirmation should include a positive, present-tense statement of belief. Often, clients may challenge the instruction to repeat or hold a positive affirmation by saying, "but I *don't* accept or believe in myself." Encouraging clients to continue with the affirmation statement despite disbelief and doubts, when accompanied by acupressure point tapping, seems to help them settle into awareness and calm. This is similar to the concept of a positive override to negative thoughts and emotion. Rick Hanson (2009) expands on importance of internalizing the positive in his discussion on the broad negativity bias of memory. Hanson describes typical brain function as having a negative bias toward states of vigilance, of frequent scanning for danger, and of reactive and responsive attendance to unpleasant experiences and memories. According to Hanson, the brain is "like Velcro for negative experiences and Teflon for positive ones" (p. 68).

Thus, the use of positive affirmations, including repeatedly calling up positive images and holding these simultaneously with the negative memory, may, over time, create a shift that allows the positive to seep in, ultimately creating new neural and memory pathways. The field of positive psychology focuses on similar concepts including cultivating of thoughts of gratitude. Robert Emmons and colleagues (Emmons & Mishra, 2012) from the University of California at Davis have researched the concept of gratitude. Regarding the positive mental health benefits of incorporating a sense of gratitude, Emmons states, "The evidence strongly supports the supposition that gratitude promotes adaptive coping and personal growth" (p. 250). A creative tool for helping clients to promote adaptive coping includes keeping a daily gratitude journal. This simple task can be used as adjunct to regular trauma therapy. In the therapist's office, a container holding blank journals in various sizes, shapes, and covers can be presented to clients, allowing clients to select a journal and begin to reflect on gratitude and refocus on positive memories and experience. A simple concept and technique like positive affirmations, when included as a part of trauma therapy, may help clients shift toward positive, bring healing changes in the brain and a new sense of well-being.

Case Example

Sarah is a 39-year-old woman coming to counseling to learn skills to cope with chronic state of anxiety. Her main triggers occur around her relationship with her spouse, as she works through feelings about a past incident of husband's infidelity combined with his current job requirements of being away from home for extended periods. Her husband had asked Sarah to fly to meet and stay with him at his job site. Sarah very much wanted to make this trip and opportunity to be with her husband, but the thought of flying to meet him filled her with nearly intolerable levels of anxiety. In session, Sarah was taught the basic protocol of Emotional Freedom Technique (or EFT), also called Tapping. She practiced and learned EFT and noticed how it helped her feel a measurable reduction in her anxiety levels.

She used tapping prior to boarding the plane, at different moments throughout the flight, and before her plane touched down and she met her husband at the gate. At a later session, Sarah recounted how she made it through what she had thought would be unbearable, and how she continues to use tapping when she notices her elevated levels of anxiety.

Nutrition, Sleep Hygiene, Exercise

With an eye turned toward trauma assessment and treatment, therapists may miss the opportunity for trauma interventions at a basic level. Behavioral health assessments for conditions like depression usually include inquiry of recent activity level, recent weight loss or weight gain, and habits of sleep. Initial intake for clients with PTSD should include similar assessments of physiological functioning. At minimum, questions regarding clients' most recent date of annual physical exam or doctor's visit should be asked. Psychoeducation given to clients can provide neuroscience-based rationale for physical interventions aimed to improve nutritional status, improve sleep, and encourage exercise.

Nutrition

In the rush to discover new methods (usually pharmaceutical) for treatment of mental health conditions, basic and fundamental modalities are often overlooked. Dietary interventions and the access to healthy, nutrient-rich foods may be an intervention both preventative and supportive. Ironically, a shift in dietary habits for many Americans from agrarian, fresh from the local farm to packaged, processed, and convenient has often resulted in less than optimal levels of nutrients available for metabolic functioning. Even as many people seek important information and instructions for better nutritional health and functioning, many sources of nutritional information may provide conflicting information. For example, many adopted the recommendations to remove or decrease high intake of dietary fats and oils. However, such a diet that is low fat or "fat free" and promoted as being healthy and a way to avoid obesity, can actually be dangerous and harmful, particularly for young children. The brain itself is the organ in the body that contains the most fat, being comprised of 60% fat (Chang et al., 2009). It is crucial for the best type of dietary fat to be included in the diet to assist in proper brain development, for repair following injury, and for ongoing optimal functioning. Particularly for infants and toddlers with their rapidly developing brain and connection-building neurons, an intake of proper fats is crucial and sets the stage for lifelong optimal mental health functioning.

So what are the ideal types of fat necessary for proper brain development and mental health functioning? There are four types of fat: trans fats, saturated fats, monounsaturated fats, and polyunsaturated fats. These each have different chemical makeup. Trans fats and saturated fats should be avoided. These are the fats that tend to be more solid at room temperature. General guidelines frequently recommend that a focus on Omega 3 type of fatty acids is beneficial. Omega 3 fatty acids are found in certain fish such as salmon or in fish oil supplements. The American Heart Association website has an individual fat intake calculator that can help to better adhere to guidelines for daily dietary fat intake (www.heart.org).

While most dietary recommendations are framed in the perspective of heart health, the dietary requirements for healthy brain and nervous system functioning should not be overlooked. Adequate vitamin intake including vitamin D, water-soluble B vitamin, and immune system–boosting vitamin C are particularly important for proper function-ing and good health.

Vitamin D, also called Calcitriol, was identified as a vita-min early in the 20th century and is now recognized as a steroid-related hormone. Vitamin D has many recep-tor sites and plays a role in many aspects of the function-ing of the body, particularly functions related to calcium and phosphorus requirements in the body. An interesting fact about vitamin D is that it is best obtained either from foods eaten or by simple exposure of sunlight to the skin. The use of sunscreen, while important for prevention of skin cancer, may have been a contributing factor in the observed increased levels of vitamin D deficiency. When sunscreen effectually blocks the sunlight from the skin, the skin may be prevented from the chemical processes of converting sunlight to vitamin D. Since the body can also metabolize vitamin D through dietary intake, medical prescription supplementation may be an option for some people with vitamin D deficiency. Vitamin D levels can be tested, and physicians are increasingly requesting that lev-els be assessed as part of regular annual lab testing.

Recent studies are pointing to interesting mind–body connections between the brain and the human intesti-nal tract. The intestinal tract is sometimes even referred to as the second brain. The intestine is the only organ of the body having its own nervous system, with an esti-mated 100 million closely connected neurons within the intestinal wall. The gut and the brain communicate back and forth by means of the nervous system via the vagus nerve, through neurohormones and neurotrans-mitters, and through the immune system. There are an estimated 100 trillion microbes that make their home in the human intestinal tract. A most fascinating fact is that these microbes outnumber our human body cells 10 to 1. This vast internal ecosystem is known as the microbiome.

Gut bacteria help regulate digestion, influence metabolism, create and utilize vitamins, extract key nutrients from our food, and exert influence on the immune system. Finally, the bacteria help produce neurochemicals that the brain uses for memory, mood, and learning functions. An estimated 95% of the body's serotonin is manufactured in the gut (Carpenter, 2012). Attention is being paid to potential beneficial actions of certain bacteria known collectively as probiotics. Research is showing that increasing probiotic bacteria levels may help to reduce cortisol levels. Reductions of chronically elevated cortisol levels has many positive health benefits, including slowing of the heart rate, lowering blood pressure, and producing a positive brain effect on mood, motivation, and fear responses. Others studies have identified gut microbes which actively secrete the neurotransmitter GABA (Davidson, 2014).

In 2007, the International Human Microbiome Project was started through the National Institutes of Health to study the microbiome in human health. Even as more research becomes available for review, clinicians may still make general nutritional recommendations such as maintaining a nutrient-rich diet, including probiotic sources such as yogurt with active cultures, and taking adequate vitamins including vitamin D and the B-complex vitamins, both crucial for healthy nervous system functioning.

Sleep Hygiene

An estimated 30 to 40 million Americans have difficulty falling asleep, staying asleep, or returning to sleep after early waking. Insomnia is a frequent symptom of many mental health conditions such as depression, bipolar disorder, and anxiety. Nightmares that disrupt sleep are common in PTSD. Sleep disturbances common in trauma may include nightmares, sleep-onset complaints, late night awakening,

and an increase in a sleep disturbance called sleep paralysis. In a review of research on connections between sleep
disturbances and PTSD, Orr and Lettieri (2011) found
that sleep disturbances that are common after experiencing a traumatic event may go on to become a pattern and
set the stage for the sleep disorder criteria as described in
DSM-5 (American Psychiatric Association, 2013). Sleep disturbances also may coincide with development of mood
disorders. Research is also exploring whether sleep disorders may have an influence on natural resiliency and of
themselves be a possible predisposing factor for PTSD. Further studies are looking at possible associations between
presence of sleep disturbances as a predictive indicator for
severity of PTSD.

Sleep disorders are only a part of larger neuroscience
research attention around circadian rhythm functions
and connections to health including mental health.
Roughly one third of our lives are spent in sleep; however in reality there is a constant ebb and flow of body
activity throughout each day that influences all the functions of the body and nervous system. This biological
clock is influenced by endogenous functions within the
body and through interaction with environmental stimuli such as light. At the University of Oxford researcher
Russell Foster is studying possible connections between
circadian rhythm disruptions and mental illness. Foster
and colleagues discovered the presence of a new type
of neuron located in the retina in the back of the eye
(Foster et al., 1991) This cell, called a photosensitive
retinal ganglion cell, is found to exist in the eye alongside functioning rod cells involved in sight processes in
low levels of light, and cone cells, which allow for color
vision and the higher visual acuity required for vision.
Detection of the presence of light upon retinal ganglion
cells send signals back to an area in the hypothalamus

called the suprachiasmatic nucleus. Alongside this area of the hypothalamus is a small gland called the pineal gland. This gland of the endocrine system was one of the last glands discovered to exist in the body. As described in Chapter 2, one of many functions of the hypothalamus is regulation of the sleep–wake cycle. This includes signaling a release of neurohormones, which results in complex patterns of interaction that determines levels of alertness or rest. Upon detection of low levels of light on the retina and signals sent to the hypothalamus, the pineal gland is stimulated to release melatonin. There is complexity in the interactions of various neurotransmitters and neurohormones relating to sleep–wake cycles and the maintenance of an overriding state called sleep–wake homeostasis. Other neurotransmitters are joined in a ballet of interactions influencing sleep–wake homeostasis, including histamine, serotonin, glutamate, dopamine, norepinephrine, acetylcholine, and orexin. Orexin (also called hypocretin) was discovered in 1996 and was found to be an important neurohormonal factor in regulating alertness, arousal, and wakefulness (Ebrahim et al., 2002). Orexin is also involved in appetite regulation. Emerging research from Uppsala University (2015), suggests that PTSD with an accompanying alteration of brain anatomy and function may be due in part to an imbalance between neurochemical signaling systems in the brain specifically of serotonin and substance P. (Uppsala University, 2015).

The trauma therapist can provide education, referral, and support to clients as they begin to address sleep-related concerns. Basic sleep hygiene habits can be established, beginning with paying attention to factors that may inhibit sleep. For example, clients can be encouraged to keep a sleep diary to provide a record of baseline sleep activity and possible sleep issues. Adolescent clients in particular often sleep next to cell phones and electronic devices, or use such devices in hours just prior to sleep. Recent studies suggest that light emission from electronic devices may disrupt release of melatonin and alter circadian rhythm functions. Therapists can encourage young clients to 'unplug' from devices at night and avoid use of computers or other devices several hours before sleep. A report by the American Academy of Pediatrics mentions common factors related to sleep disorders in adolescents and young adults (Owens, 2014). These include factors related to electronic devices, an increase in consumption of caffeine, and differences with adolescent hormonal patterns of melatonin release and circadian patterns.

Across the life span there also may be sleep pattern changes and differing issues related to disrupted sleep affecting mood, cognition, and functioning. It is beyond the scope of this book to discuss these issues in depth; however, the therapist should have a working knowledge of sleep disorders, as well as access to referral sources for sleep disorder specialists when necessary. The therapist working in trauma should always include assessment of sleep functions as fundamental to treatment planning.

Exercise

Creative approaches to therapy for trauma should include prescription for exercise and the incorporation of movement-related activity into daily life. Exercise is often overlooked by mental health professionals as an integral part of mental health and trauma treatment plans. Exercise has been shown to help reduce anxiety, depression, and negative moods while increasing self-esteem and improving cognitive functioning. Exercise increases the circulation of blood to the brain and influences the HPA axis with a resulting decrease in level of reactivity to stress (Shanna et al., 2006). Physical exercise has also been shown to increase neurogenesis within the hippocampus and to improve spatial learning (Ming & Song, 2011).

A prescription for exercise is common for clients in my office. Specifically, I recommend starting with 10 minutes (minimum) of mindful walking each day, paying particular attention to the cross-body bipedal motion of walking. Simple focus on rhythm of right arm swings with left leg step, and alternating, encourages cross-body motion and right brain–left brain integration. During walking, clients should allow direct sunlight to fall on exposed skin of face or body. This has the added benefit of providing an increase in production of vitamin D in the body, with its own accompanying benefits to mental health (of course, a nice walk on a cloudy day with a warm, gentle rain may have calming, sensory-soothing benefits as well). Other exercise modalities such as strength training and weight lifting may also make a positive contribution to mental health functioning. Running and other exercise has been found to enhance neurofunctioning in three specific ways: through a rapid increase in production of BDNF (brain-derived neurotrophic factor) in the hippocampus following exercise; an increase in serotonin levels, and an increase in angiogenesis (creation of blood vessels) in the brain that in turn provide increased oxygenation to the brain. Researcher van Praag (2009) mentions that the brain benefits of exercise can be further enhanced by dietary addition of omega fatty acids and plant-based foods. A brain healing approach to trauma may include a prescription of exercise, and increased attention to diet as early and standard objectives for treatment.

Nature Therapies

Many times, the therapy office might not be the ideal environment for trauma healing for a client. There is often a profound disconnect between the natural world and people today. Particularly among youth, little time is spent outdoors or other inside pursuits take precedence. Some studies are beginning to suggest that literal connection with the earth is healing and important for well-being. In the book *Earthing*, authors Ober et al. (2010) describe ion and energy exchange between person and earth when people remove shoes and sit or walk upon the (un-concrete) ground. What a soothing prescription it can be for clients to be instructed to take off their shoes and walk gently upon the ground.

Wilderness experiences are often recommended to help remove a person from habitual patterns of thought and surround them with novel sensory experiences as found in nature. Connection with earth can also be found in therapeutic gardening. Bringing the elements into the therapy office is also helpful. Water in fountains, therapy stones, the flame of a candle, seashells, or artwork and photography with a nature focus can be initially soothing to clients. The element of water in particular has been shown to be calming to a dysregulated nervous system.

In his recent book called *Blue Minds*, marine biologist Wallace J. Nichols describes how closeness to water in many different forms can be beneficial to our mental, physical, and emotional health. Nichols (2014) describes how regular exposure to nature, and more specifically to water, allows the mind to relax and *not* to hold onto directed and alert focus states. Nichols mentions the work of psychologist Stephen Kaplan and colleagues at the University of Michigan who study the interactive effects of nature on brain functioning. Nature is filled with many intriguing and interesting stimuli that fill the mind with what Kaplan calls "soft fascination" or a state of effortless awareness and gentle curiosity (Kaplan, 1995). Further, this awareness occurs in a bottom-up manner, which seems to then allow space for top-down, finely focused attention and encourage moments for rest and rejuvenation.

Case Example

Marie is a 14-year-old struggling with depression and social anxiety disorder. Her anxiety levels are increasingly elevated, particularly around school settings as she begins to have poor school attendance and an increasing sense of isolation and disconnection. The therapist initially works with Marie to help establish the counseling office as a safe, calming place where she can learn tools for managing anxiety and soothing her activated nervous system. In one midsummer early evening session, Marie requested, "Can we please just go for a walk instead of talking?" Welcoming the suggestion, the therapist led Marie out to the park adjoining the counselor's office building. This park was full of tall shaded cottonwoods and green grassy areas. Marie seemed to gain new spring to her step and a softening of her shoulders and face.

Playfully, she encouraged the therapist to accompany her to the playground area where she stepped onto an adult-sized old fashioned seesaw. (This proved a bit of a feat for the therapist in business attire and high-heeled shoes.) Shoes were removed, and the rest of session time consisted of connection with nature, the balance of the seesaw, and groundedness. Marie began to talk of the sadness and loneliness of her social isolation, and the therapist became a container for her story and an encourager for reconnection in her life.

These positive, creative counseling interventions are guiding therapists to new, holistic, and integrative approaches to treatment.

References

American Music Therapy Association. (n.d.). What is music therapy? (retrieved March 26, 2016 from www.musictherapy. org/about/musictherapy/)

American Psychiatric Association. (2013). *Diagnostic and statistical manual of mental disorders* (5th ed.). Washington, DC: Author. Text citation: (American Psychiatric Association, 2013).

Bensimon, M., Amir, D., & Wolf, Y. (2008). Drumming through trauma: Music therapy with post traumatic soldiers. *The Arts in Psychotherapy*, 35, 34–48.

Benson, H. (1975). Steps to elicit the relaxation response. (retrieved April 30, 2015 from www.relaxationresponse.org/ steps/)

Bernardi, L., Porta, C., Casucci,G., Balsamo, R., Bernardi, N.F., Fogari, R., & Sleight, P. (2009). Dynamic interactions between musical, cardiovascular, and cerebral rhythms in humans. *Circulation*, 119:3171–3180, 19546392. (retrieved April 22, 2015 from www.medscape.com)

Carpenter, S. (2012). That gut feeling: With a sophisticated neural network transmitting messages from trillions of bacteria, the brain in your gut exerts powerful influences over the one in your head. *American Psychological Association*, 43(8), 1–4.

Chang, C., Ke, D., & Chen, J. (2009). Essential fatty acids and human brain. *Acta Neurologica Taiwanic*, 18(4). (retrieved March 30, 2016 from www.researchgate.net)

Collie, K., Backos, A., Malchiodi, C., & Spiegel, D. (2006). Art therapy for combat related PTSD: Recommendations for research and practice. *Art Therapy: Journal of the American Art Therapy Association*, 23(4), 157–164.

Davidson, J. (2014). The psychobiotic revolution: It may be possible to relieve anxiety and depression solely by manipulating bacteria in the gut. *Psychology Today*, March/April, 2014.

DeAngelis, T. (2008). PTSD treatments grow in evidence, effectiveness: Several psychological interventions help to significantly reduce post-traumatic stress disorder, say new guidelines. *American Psychological Association*, 39(1), 40.

Ebrahim, I. O., Howard, R. S., Kopelman, M. D., Sharief, M. K., & Williams, A. J. (2002). The hypocretin/orexin system.

Journal of the Royal Society of Medicine, 95(5), 227–230. (retrieved December 8, 2015 from www.ncbi.nlm.nih.gov/pmc/articles/ PMC12796731/)

Emmons, R. A., & Mishra, A. (2012). Why gratitude enhances well-being: What we know, what we need to know. In Sheldon, K., Kashdan, T., & Steger, M.F. (Eds.), *Designing the future of positive psychology: Taking stock and moving forward*. New York: Oxford University Press. [pdf] (retrieved March 30, 2016 from http://emmons.faculty.ucdavis.edu/wp- content/uploads/ sites/90/2015/08/2011_2–16_Sheldon_Chapter-16-11. pdf)

Feinstein, D. (2012, September). Rapid treatment of PTSD: Why psychological exposure with acupoint tapping may be effective. *Psychotherapy: Theory, Research, Practice, Training. American Psychological Association*, 47(3), 385–402. (retrieved March 29, 2016 from http://dx.doi.org/10.1037/a0021171)

Feinstein, D. (2012). Acupoint stimulation in treating psychological disorders: Evidence of efficacy. Review of General Psychology. Advance online publication. doi:10.1037/a0028602

Follette, V., Palm, K.M., & Pearson, A.N. (2006). Mindfulness and trauma: Implications for treatment. *Journal of Rationale-Emotive and Cognitive- Behavior Therapy*, 24(1), 45–61, doi: 10.1007/s 10942-006-0025-2

Foster, R.G., Provencio, I., Hudson, D., Fiske, S., Grip, W., & Menaker, M. (1991). Circadian photoreception in the retinally degenerate mouse (rd/rd). *Journal of Comparative Physiology A*, 169(1), 39–50. doi: 10.1007/BF00198171. PMID 1941717

Friedman, B.H., & Thayer, J.F. (1998). Autonomic balance revisited: Panic anxiety and heart rate variability. *Journal of Psychosomatic Research*, 44(1), 133–151.

Grand, D. (2013). *Brainspotting: The revolutionary new therapy for rapid and effective change*. Boulder, CO: Sounds True.

Hanley, K. (2015). A beginners guide to eight major styles of yoga: A brief look at different approaches to yoga and which suits your needs best. (retrieved April 2015 from www.life. gaiam.com/article/beginners-guide-8-major-styles-yoga)

Hanson, R. (2009). *Buddha's brain: The practical neuroscience of happiness, love & wisdom/Rick Hanson with Richard Mendius*. Oakland, CA: New Harbinger Publications, Inc.

Henderson, P., Rosen, D., & Mascaro, N. (2007). Empirical study on the healing nature of mandalas. *Psychology of Aesthetics, Creativity, and the Arts*, 1(3), 148–154.

Jahnke, R., Larkey, L., Rogers, C., Etnier, J., & Lin, F. (2010). A comprehensive review of health benefits of qigong and tai chi. *American Journal of Health Promotion*, July–August, 2010, 24(6), e1–e25. doi: 10.4278/ajhp.08103-LIT-248

Jung, C.G. (1965). *Memories, dreams, reflections*. In Jaffe, Aniela (ed.), Winston, Richard & Winston, Clara (Trans.) (pp. 195–196). New York: Random House (retrieved August 2015 from http://creatingmandalas.com/psychology-of-the-mandala)

Kaplan, S. (1995). The restorative benefits of nature: Toward an integrative framework. *Journal of Environmental Psychology*, 15 (3), 169–182. (retrieved March 30, 2016 from http://willsull. net/resources/KaplanS1995.pdf)

Levitin, D.J. (2006). *This is your brain on music: The science of a human obsession*. New York: Penguin Group.

Malchiodi, C.A. (2005). *Expressive therapies: History, theory, and practice*. New York: Guilford Press.

Ming, G., & Song, H. (2011). Neurogenesis in the adult mammalian brain: Significant answers and significant questions. *Neuron*, 70(4), 687–702. (retrieved May 11, 2015 from *ncbi. nlm.nih.gov*)

National Geographic. (2015). Behind the mask: Revealing the trauma of war. (retrieved March 30, 2016 from www.national geographic.com/healing-soldiers/)

National Public Radio. (2015). The search for well-being: Treating the whole person in the new health care era. A primer on integrative medicine. (retrieved April 12, 2015 from www. humanmedia.org National Public Radio International)

Nichols, W.J. (2014). *Blue minds: The surprising science that shows how being near, in, on, or under water can make you happier, healthier, more connected, and better at what you do*. New York: Little, Brown and Company.

Novotny, S., & Kravitz, L. (2007). The science of breathing. *IDEA Fitness Journal*, 4(2), 36–43.

Ober, C., Sinatra, S.T., & Zucker, M. (2010). *Earthing: The most important health discovery ever?* Laguna Beach, CA: Basic Health Publications, Inc.

Ogden, P., Pain, C., & Fisher, J. (2006). A sensorimotor approach to the treatment of trauma and dissociation. *Psychiatric Clinics of North America,* 29, 262–279.

Orr, N.H., & Lettieri, C.J. (2011, March 16). Sleep disturbances and posttraumatic stress disorder. *Medscape.*

Owens, J., American Academy of Pediatrics. (2014). Technical report: Insufficient sleep in adolescents and young adults: An update on causes and consequences. (retrieved March 30, 2016 from www.pediatrics.org/cgi/doi/10.1542/peds *2014–1696*)

Parnell, L. (2008). *Tapping in: A step-by-step guide to activating your healing resources through bilateral stimulation.* Boulder, CO: Sounds True, Inc.

Payne, P., Levine, P.A., & Crane-Godreau, M.A. (2015). Somatic experiencing: Using interoception and proprioception as core elements of trauma therapy. *Frontiers in Psychology,* 6(Article 93), 1–18. doi: 10.3389/fpsyg.2015.00093

Pennebaker, J.W., & Seagal, J.D. (1999). Forming a story: The health benefits of narrative. *Journal of Clinical Psychology,* 55 (10), 1243–1254.

Powers, S. (2008). *Insight yoga: An innovative synthesis of traditional yoga, meditation, and eastern approaches for healing and well-being.* Boston: Shambhala Publications, Inc.

Sakai, C. S., Connolly, S. M., & Oas, P. (2010). Treatment of PTSD in Rwandan genocide survivors using thought field therapy. *International Journal of Emergency Mental Health,* 12(1), 41–50.

Shanna, A., Madaan, V., & Frederick, D.P. (2006). Exercise for mental health. *Primary Care Companion to the Journal of Clinical Psychiatry,* 8(2), 106. (retrieved April 25, 2015 from ncbi.nlm.nih.gov)

Siegel, D.J. (1999). *The developing mind.* New York: The Guilford Press.

Siegel, D.J. (2010). *Mindsight: The new science of personal transformation.* New York: Random House.

Solomon, R.M., & Shapiro, F. (2008). EMDR and the adaptive information processing model: Potential mechanisms of change. *Journal of EMDR Practice and Research,* 2(4), 315–325.

Uppsala University. (2015, December 1). Posttraumatic stress disorder reveals an imbalance between signalling systems in the brain. *Medical News Today.* (retrieved December 4, 2015 from www.medicalnewstoday.com/releases/303359.php)

van der Kolk, B.A. (2015). Yoga as a complementary treatment for chronic PTSD. (retrieved April 2015 from www.trauma center.org/research/yoga_study.php)

Van Praag, H. (2009). Exercise and the brain: Something to chew on. *Trends in Neurosciences*, 32(5), 283–290. doi: 10.1016/j. tins.2008.12.007 (retrieved March 28, 2016 from www.ncbi. nih.gov/pmc/articles/PMC2680508)

Visualization. (n.d.). In *Collins dictionary.* (retrieved March 27, 2016 from Collinsdictionary.com/dictionary/English/visualization)

Worwood, V.A. (1996). The fragrant mind: Aromatherapy for personality, mind, mood, and emotion. Novato, CA: New World Library.

10

TRAUMA, THE BRAIN, AND THE FUTURE

The room is crowded and noisy; people gather around emergency personnel waiting for instructions on returning to what might remain of their homes. A woman sits alone near a wall, a detached and distant look in her eyes. Children play a pickup game of tag, while others cling to their parents. The disaster mental health volunteers have a quick briefing in the corner of the room. "Look to the community members to assist the outreach team. They know the community resources," says one. "We just got a new shipment of water so should be good to go," says another. "There is a woman sitting alone with a twenty-mile stare. Maybe someone can reach out to her?" Walking out toward the crowd, the team leader says,

> Remember, reactions you see may be considered normal reactions to an abnormal situation.

This book has talked about the brain and discoveries of how the brain functions and interacts with the world both outside and in. Aided by advances in technology, discoveries in neuroscience and the brain are occurring at an unprecedented pace. With every answer comes many new questions. While the tendency may be to focus on psychopathology and on discussion of diagnostic criteria, the experience of trauma is personal and unique for each person. Just as every human brain is complex, with neural connections vast as the universe, researchers and clinicians recognize how little they know. The observation that a majority of people do not go on to develop PTSD after trauma may give pause, as we to try to determine instead how the brain will adapt and recover from damage or respond to trauma with resilience. The remarkable manner in which the brain can recover from injury both inspires and pushes toward ways to prevent brain and spinal cord injury and disease of the nervous system, as well as to support cultural and public health interventions for prevention of trauma affecting individuals, families, communities, and cultures, and to mitigate negative effects of disaster and trauma.

New Findings in Neuroscience

In the meantime, research in neuroscience is looking not just at regeneration of neural cellular functioning, but at earlier processes related to the immediate cellular responses to injury. Not only neuroscience, but research in general medicine has discovered connections between inflammation, the immune system, and processes that may lead to chronic bodily illness and disease. Possible links have been discovered between immune response with inflammation and the onset of chronic illness such as heart disease, autoimmune disorders, Alzheimer's disease, and others.

The central nervous system is known to have a protective mechanism called the blood–brain barrier, which protects the brain by preventing harmful pathogens or large molecular substances from traveling from the bloodstream of the body into the brain. New discoveries suggest that the immune system response of inflammation may play a role in neurodegenerative diseases such as depression, anxiety, and other mental health–related conditions.

Inflammation is actually a necessary part of the body's process of healing. The inflammatory response on the cellular level is influenced by a protein substance called cytokine. Cytokines have been shown to increase communication between cells and to direct immune cells to areas of injury, infection, or trauma. The actions of cytokines play a role in the inflammatory immune response. The inflammatory response includes increased temperature and swelling at the site of injury, which helps to kill bacteria and foreign invaders, and surrounding or immobilizing foreign invaders, which allows the immune system clean-up crew to process or remove the harmful threat. Another area of research focus involves the normal mechanisms of cellular metabolism. There are ongoing processes of both cellular energy use and maintenance (or allostasis), as well as cellular death (or apoptosis). Energy utilization within the cell occurs within the part of a cell known as the mitochondria. The mitochondria of the cell is the storage and production site for the energy used to move our bodies and to maintain proper cell growth and energy production. It accomplishes this through a complex process and utilization of oxygen through the production of a substance called ATP (adenosine triphosphate). In the body, substances known as oxidants are formed as a normal by-product of aerobic (or oxygen-requiring) metabolism. However, an overabundance of harmful oxidants, called oxidative stress, may be produced under harmful physiological conditions and stress. Continuing exposure to certain stressors can result in inflammation in body and brain that may result in many of the chronic illness conditions including heart disease, cancer, and diabetes. For example, there is a connection between inflammation around the teeth and gums and heart disease.

The possible role of inflammatory processes in the central nervous system is being eyed for associations with behavioral health conditions such as major depressive disorder, anxiety, and other conditions. Recent research (Dantzer et al., 2008) has focused on the typical behavioral responses to infections such as malaise, low energy, and listlessness. These behaviors are referred to as 'sickness behaviors.' It was thought that these symptoms were simply a typical or common behavioral response to infection in the body. These behavioral symptoms are now being studied as a consequence of the cytokines responding to peripheral infection in the body signaling an immune or inflammatory response in the brain. Inflammation occurs when cells are damaged by invasion of bacteria, during trauma or injury, or by exposure to toxic substances. When cells are damaged they may release small protein molecule substances such as cytokines, which act like a chemical message delivery service. Cytokines send messages to nearby cells and activate other immune cells to clean up or mitigate the damaged cells. The small size of the cytokine molecule allows it to travel across the blood–brain barrier. This is believed to occur through the hypothalamus-pituitary-adrenal axis. Therefore, inflammation occurring in the body as a response to infection or illness or exposure to chemicals or environmental toxins can travel along pathways crossing the blood–brain barrier into the brain. Also, traumatic brain injury can cause damage to brain cells directly through subsequent inflammatory processes after the injury. Specific neural cells involved in inflammatory and reparative efforts following injury include glial cells located throughout the brain. Increases in brain cytokines signaling appears to impair learning and memory consolidation and may even be related to increased susceptibility to depression. Such research is pointing to new brain–body–immune system approaches to understanding depression and other behavioral health–physical health connections.

Other new research is exploring the actions of various neurotransmitters and amino acids within the brain. For years the treatment for depression has focused on the actions of serotonin and dopamine in the brain. However, for many people antidepressants do not seem to be helpful at relieving depression, and for those who may be helped, antidepressants often take weeks to begin to work. Additionally, there can be undesirable side effects with antidepressant use. New attention is looking at possible malfunctioning of the neurotransmitter system for glutamate and GABA in conditions such as certain depressive disorders, panic disorders, schizophrenia, and even in suicidal clients (Sharpley, 2009). There is new information about potential treatments for hospitalized suicidal patients using the anesthetic called ketamine, which seems to impact the neurotransmitter glutamate within the brain (McMillen, 2014). Additionally, individual genetic testing is beginning to point to an ability to predict which type of psychotropic medication might be most effective and specific for each individual. These are amazing times for neuroscience research and the clinical applications of research findings. In trauma treatment, support and adaptations from ancient concepts such as mindfulness, yoga, and other practices are gaining credence from research findings and pointing to new ways to approach treatment.

Genetic research and related new discoveries are poised to introduce changes in treatment of mental illness in other ways as well. The new field of pharmacogenomics is studying how an individual's genome might affect her response to commonly prescribed psychotropic medications (Mrazek, 2010). Specifically, pharmacogenomics hopes to be able to predict who might have adverse effects or side effects when given certain medications. While medication management has been the common medical approach to treatment of depression and anxiety, making antidepressants among the most highly prescribed medications worldwide, only a third to half of patients have a good initial response to these drugs. Successful treatment is even more elusive with each medication trial and failure. Advances in pharmacogenomics have pinpointed several genes that encode for enzymes known as P450 (CYP). These enzymes help to metabolize or process most drugs for use in the body, including drugs affecting neurotransmitters and systemic or neurological functioning (Harrison, 2015). Identification of the presence of various CYPs may predict whether a person might benefit from treatment with a specific psychotropic medication, or if that substance would be poorly processed, building up in levels in the blood or in the brain and resulting in adverse reactions or side effects. Currently, a simple cheek swab sample may be obtained and sent for gene analysis. Individual genetic coding may aid in determination of targeted treatment matching optimal medication for each individual (Elsevier, 2013). With implications for treatment of mood disorders and more, there is nevertheless controversy over widespread clinical use of this technology. There are ethical, economic, and other considerations for use of pharmacogenomics at this time. Still, this new technology is available and slowly becoming integrated on the clinic level. It is important that the counselor be aware of and learn about pharmacogenomics so that they may better respond to clients with questions regarding these options being presented to them.

Case Example

John is a 67-year-old retired veteran coming to counseling for treatment of depression. He has suffered from depression off and on for a number of years. His psychiatrist has prescribed various antidepressants over the years, and none seem to have been positively effective in the treatment of his depression. John reported to the counselor that his doctor is recommending that he have genomic testing to point the direction for the most effective medication for treatment. John reports that the doctor explained this to him, but stated to the counselor that he feels unsure and a little uneasy about giving a saliva sample for analysis of his DNA. He expressed concerns primarily about possible misuse of this information and his hesitations regarding who might have access to his personal health information. The counselor listened carefully and gave validation for John as he expressed these concerns. The counselor encouraged John to discuss these concerns with his physician to obtain information and instruction to his satisfaction. The counselor sought ethical guidelines regarding such genomic testing and consulted with a specialist in genetic counseling. At a later session, John reported that he told his doctor that he had elected not to have genome testing at this time, and had worked with his physician on developing a new plan for the pharmacological treatment for his depression.

Final mention of current neuroscience and trauma field research is looking into the occurrence and impact of trauma reflected within the expression of our genes, and at new neuroscience technologies poised to change the way we look at treatment for trauma.

Neuroplasticity and the ability of brain cells to rewire and reassemble have changed how we look at trauma recovery. The age-old question of nature versus nurture is being answered in surprising ways. The field of epigenetics informs us that while the genetic code found in DNA may not be changed structurally, stress or environmental factors may influence how unique genetic code is read or expressed. Neuroscience-guided discoveries are opening new possibilities of healing or management of mental health conditions. For example, electrical excitation applied directly to the human brain became possible in the 1980s (George, 2007). Researchers showed that direct electrical stimulation applied in specific regions of the brain can result in behavioral or functional changes within the brain. This discovery allowed surgeons to better identify and preserve healthy brain tissue during surgery and to hone in on precise removal of brain tumors or disease-affected areas. Recently, pacemakers similar to the cardiac pacemaker can be implanted in the chest with wires and electrodes leading to target areas of the brain. This shows promise for treatment to alleviate troubling symptoms of Parkinson's and other neurological disorders. A similar approach called vagus nerve stimulation (VNS) applies intermittent electrical stimulation of the vagus nerve. Currently, VNS is being used to lessen frequency or severity of epileptic seizures. Further research is seeking to discover if VNS is helpful in alleviating conditions of severe depression or anxiety. Other neuroscience research may provide direction on identifying certain individual genetic markers that, when present, may help identify which antidepressant to prescribe and utilize for individualized treatment of depression.

Knowledge and understanding of various functioning regions of the brain has developed in tandem with new technologies such as real-time functional magnetic resonance imaging (rtfMRI) and electroencephalogram (EEG). These noninvasive technologies can provide neurofeedback to individuals who can learn to self-regulate brain functioning and behavioral responses. This knowledge has suggested specificity for treatment applications as they target specific functional areas or interconnected networks within the brain. This opens new treatment strategies for self-regulation and neuromodulation of brain functioning. One new treatment strategy includes an increasing use of magnetic brain stimulation. Repetitive transcranial magnetic stimulation (TMS) is a noninvasive treatment that delivers magnetic pulses to specific brain areas. Transcranial magnetic stimulation is delivered through a coil-like device placed near the surface of the scalp. This device delivers directed magnetic currents through the scalp and skull that can excite or inhibit neural electrical processes in cortical areas of the brain (Wassermann & Zimmermann, 2012). According to a guideline review by Rossi et al. and the Safety of TMS Consensus Group (2009), transcranial magnetic stimulation has been noted in literature for various clinical uses and treatment for neurological diseases such as Parkinson's disease and epilepsy, and for psychiatric disorders such as depression, obsessive-compulsive disorder, and PTSD. Current research points to possible use of rTMS for therapeutic treatment of addictions such as cocaine addiction, by targeting areas of the dorsolateral prefrontal cortex with magnetic pulses. Results are suggesting that reductions in craving and decreased use can occur with treatment (MedlinePlus, 2015) The trauma-informed counselor should educate and increase awareness of up-to-date research around these and other potential new treatment options for their trauma clients.

These and more are current examples of how neuroscience and brain discoveries are changing and influencing how we see ourselves and our interaction in the world. Of no less significance, neuroscience research points to what therapists and clients have thought all along: that engaging in therapeutic process can actually result in measurable and observable changes in the brain and in behavioral functioning. Ultimately, the therapist serves as guide and witness for his or her clients and points to a process that goes beyond reductive explanations of the brain. Hopefully we will never lose a sense of wonder about this.

References

Dantzer, R., O'Connor, J.C., Freund, G.G., Johnson, R.W., & Kelly, K.W. (2008). From inflammation to sickness and depression: When the immune system subjugates the brain. *National Review of Neuroscience*, 9(1), 46–56. doi: 10.1038/nrn2297

Elsevier. (2013, March 28). Common gene variants explain 42% of antidepressant response. *Science Daily.* (retrieved April 26, 2015 from www.sciencedaily.com/releases/2013/03/130328091730.htm)

George, M.S. (2007). Stimulating the brain. In Bloom, F.E. (Ed.), *Best of the brain: From Scientific American* (pp. 20–34). New York/Washington, DC: Dana Press.

Harrison, P. (2015, September 4). Test predicts drug response in depression, anxiety. *Medscape.* (retrieved from www.medscape.com/viewarticle/850585)

McMillen, M. (2014, September 23). Ketamine: The future of depression treatment? *WebMD Health New.* (retrieved from www.webmd.com/depression/news/20140923/ketamine-depression?print=true)

MedlinePlus. (2015, December 3). Magnetic brain stimulation might treat cocaine addiction-cravings and use decreased in pilot study. *HealthDay.* (retrieved December 4, 2015 from www.nlm.nih.gov/medlineplus/news/fullstory_156031.html)

Mrazek, D. A. (2010). Psychiatric pharmacogenomic testing in clinical practice. *Dialogues in Clinical Neuroscience*, 12(1), 69–76.

Rossi, S., Hallett, M., Rossini, P.M., Pascual-Leone, A., & The Safety of TMS Consensus Group. (2009). Safety, ethical considerations, and application guidelines for the use of transcranial magnetic stimulation in clinical practice and research. *Clinical Neurophysiology*, 120(12), 2008–2039. (retrieved March 30, 2016 from http://doi.org/10.1016/j.clinph.2009.08.016)

Sharpley, C.F. (2009). Malfunction in GABA and glutamate as pathways to depression: A review of evidence. *Clinical Medicine: Therapeutics*, Libertas Academica, 1, 1511–1519.

Wassermann, E. M., & Zimmermann, T. (2012). Transcranial magnetic brain stimulation: Therapeutic promises and scientific gaps. *Pharmacology & Therapeutics*, 133(1), 98–107. (retrieved March 30, 2016 from http://doi.org/10.1016/j.pharmthera.2011.09.003)

INDEX

Lightning Source UK Ltd.
Milton Keynes UK
UKHW020143161019
351624UK00022B/396/P